> " **WE WANT TO CHALLENGE YOU,** as we challenge ourselves, to move toward plant-based foods. We all have a responsibility to stand up for our health and the health of the planet. Let's take this stand together.
>
> **—BEYONCÉ AND JAY-Z**

> " Today, as I strive to be my best, **I MOVE TOWARD PLANTS,** I listen to Marco Borges and follow a lifestyle that truly reverses aging: *The Greenprint.*
>
> **—STEVE HARVEY**

> " **A REVOLUTIONARY MOVEMENT** that will surely inspire current and future generations to eat more plant-based foods than others in recent American history.
>
> **—DEAN ORNISH, MD,** *New York Times* bestselling author

> " **A DOABLE BLUEPRINT** packed with all the tools and resources required to finally take control of your health, transform your life, and embrace your best self. *A MUST-READ!*
>
> **—RICH ROLL,** bestselling author of *Finding Ultra* and coauthor of *The Plantpower Way*

> " **I AM RECOMMENDING** Marco Borges's *The Greenprint* to all of our patients. It is a must-have if you are ready to take control of your health.
>
> **—NEAL BARNARD, MD, FACC,** *New York Times* bestselling author

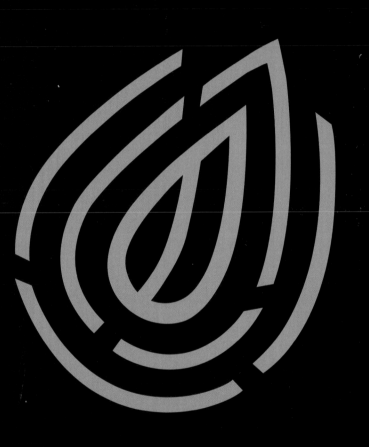

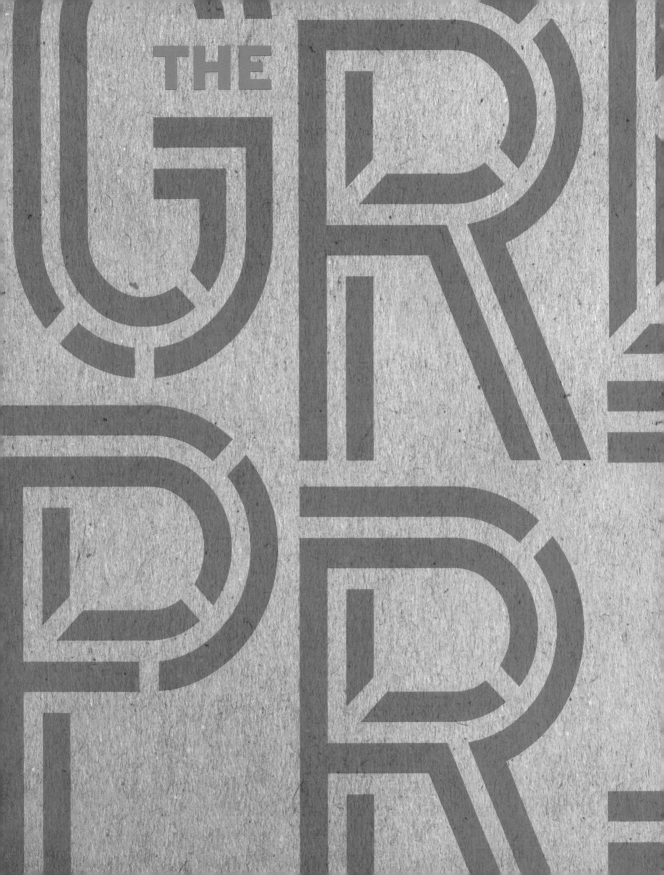

PLANT-BASED
DIET
BEST
BODY
BETTER
PLANET

MARCO BORGES

HARMONY BOOKS // NEW YORK

Published in the United States by Harmony Books,
an imprint of the Crown Publishing Group, a division of
Penguin Random House LLC, New York.
crownpublishing.com

Harmony Books is a registered trademark, and the Circle
colophon is a trademark of Penguin Random House LLC.

Library of Congress Cataloging-in-Publication Data
Names: Borges, Marco, author.
Title: The greenprint : plant-based diet, best body,
    better world / by Marco Borges.
Description: New York : Harmony Books, [2018] | Includes
    bibliographical references.
Identifiers: LCCN 2018037903 | ISBN 978-1-9848-2310-6 (hardcover)
Subjects: LCSH: Vegetarian cooking. | Cooking (Natural foods) |
    Food industry and trade—Environmental aspects. | LCGFT:
    Cookbooks.
Classification: LCC TX837 .B573 2018 | DDC 641.5/636—dc23 LC
    record available at https://lccn.loc.gov/2018037903

ISBN 978-1-9848-2310-6
Ebook ISBN 978-1-9848-2311-3

Printed in the United States of America

Cover and book design by Laura Palese Design
Photographs by Lauren Volo

10 9 8 7 6 5 4 3 2 1

First Edition

TO MY AMAZING
FAMILY AND THE
BEAUTIFUL WORLD
THEY WILL INHERIT.
WITHOUT YOU,
NOTHING IS POSSIBLE.

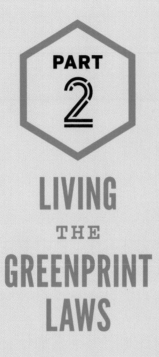

PART
2

LIVING
THE
GREENPRINT
LAWS

INTRODUCTION

BY

JAY-Z

///////

BEYONCÉ"

Having children has changed our lives more than anything else. We realize now, more than ever, that most of the things we want for ourselves we also want for the world—peace, happiness, love, prosperity, and, above all, health. We used to think of health as a diet—some worked for us, some didn't. Once we looked at health as the truth, instead of a diet, it became a mission for us to share that truth and lifestyle with as many people as possible.

We are not about promoting any one way of living your life. You decide what's best for you. What we are encouraging is for everyone to incorporate more plant-based meals into their everyday lives. As our dear friend and plant-based guru Marco always says, "The more you lean toward plants, the more you benefit."

The facts about plant-based eating are hard to ignore. The benefits of a single plant-based meal per day can have a profound impact on our health and the environment. Chronic diseases seem more prevalent than ever before—especially among those with lower income levels and less access to real food. It's not a poverty issue. It's not a minority issue. It's an all-of-us issue. The world won't change itself. *We* need to change it. A single decision by one person can affect change not only within themselves but also within their family, their community, and the planet.

We want to challenge you, as we challenge ourselves, to move toward plant-based foods. We all have a responsibility to stand up for our health and the health of the planet. Let's take this stand together. Let's spread the truth. Let's make this mission a movement. Let's become "the Greenprint."

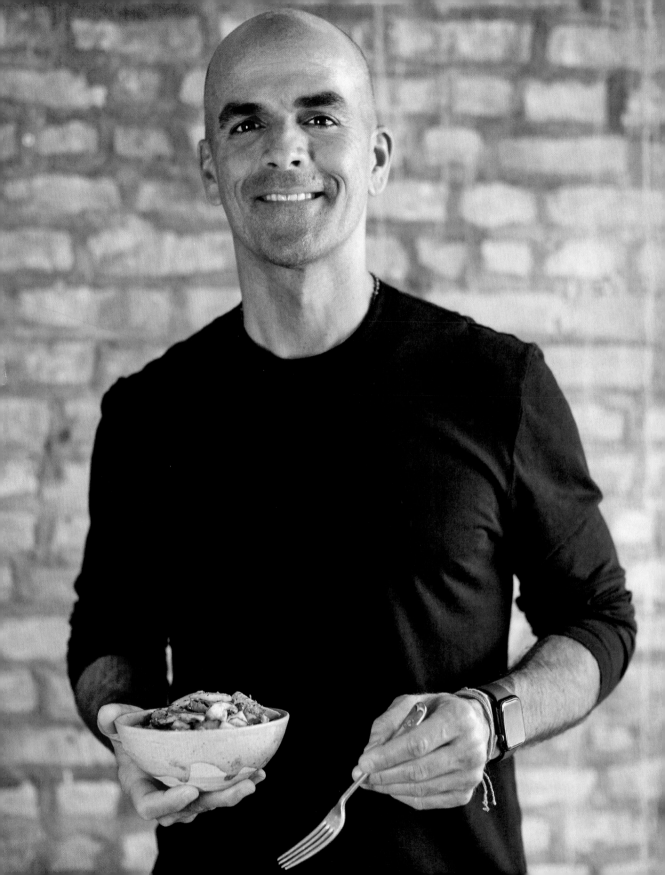

GETTING STARTED

WELCOME TO THE GREENPRINT! /////

You are about to embark on the single greatest action you can take to prevent and reverse disease, a supreme program for rapid, sustainable weight loss and improved health. It will change your life, your body, and the planet, in a revolutionary way. And it all starts with plants.

AT **ITS CORE,** the Greenprint is a revolutionary set of laws that have been created using clinical data and years of expertise that will allow you to take control of your health once and for all. As the world becomes more aware of the benefits of plant-based eating than ever before in history, *The Greenprint* is more than a book—it is a movement, and you're about to join.

As an exercise physiologist and the CEO and founder of 22 Days Nutrition, I've dedicated my life to helping people live their best lives. This means encouraging people to transition to plant-based eating so they can lose weight, prevent (and in some cases reverse) chronic disease, boost their energy, and transform their health.

Why do I do this? Because I care about you, I care about my children, and I care about their children. I want to see you live your best and healthiest life. You see, in the last hundred years, our diets have radically changed—for the worse. We've gone from eating whole foods that nourish and heal the body to eating processed junk that is high in fat, sugar, additives, toxins, and fillers yet lacks vital nutrients. We've gone from eating around 100 pounds of meat (which was raised on farms, grass fed, and free from chemicals) each year to, on average, more than 200 pounds, nearly all of it grown on factory farms and pumped full of antibiotics and hormones to satisfy the need for cheap, readily available meat. It's no wonder that, as a whole, we are the fattest and unhealthiest generation thus far.

The way we're living just isn't sustainable.

Not for us.

Not for the planet.

And that's where the Greenprint movement comes in. It offers an extraordinary plan for how to eat to get fit and healthy with foods that are greener for the earth and better for you. What is unique about the Greenprint is that it gives you the essential steps you need to start thriving on plant-based eating and take it as far as you want to go to achieve all your health and weight-loss goals. You will discover the most effective way to transform your body and your life through plant-based eating, one meal at a time. The twenty-two Greenprint laws provide plenty of advice and inspiration, and you can begin to apply them one law at a time.

Along the way, you'll find a better way of eating and living—and one that significantly contributes to the health and sustainability of the earth. You'll even be able to see tangible proof that your choices work: I'll give you a fun and easy tool to calculate your personal impact on the planet. So rest assured, you're about to go on an amazing journey with me, one that will help you live a longer, better life and make the world more livable for future generations.

Before I elaborate, I bet you're wondering, *What's a "greenprint"?*

A greenprint is a measure of the impact of our *food choices* on our weight and overall health and on our planet. For example, let's say you switch to a 100 percent plant-based diet (I hope you do). The impact—the *greenprint*—of this change on your health can be measured in years: Studies show that plant-based people, particularly if they don't smoke and drink only a little, if any, alcohol, live four to seven years longer than people whose diets include animal products. It can also be measured in positive changes in health parameters: lower blood pressure, lower blood lipids, lower blood sugar, and lower weight. With regard to weight, on average, those who consume a plant-based diet are naturally twenty pounds lighter than their meat-eating counterparts.

As for your personal greenprint on the planet, it can be colossal. You can save animals, for example. Those that are raised for human consumption do not have great lives. Even if they are raised organically and free range, they have short lives with not much freedom. If you and your family ditch meat, dairy, and eggs, you can save two hundred animals a year, according to PETA.

From an environmental standpoint, expanding your greenprint through plant-based living saves an amazing amount of energy. We're all guilty of taking our sources of energy for granted. Just 1 calorie of animal protein requires 8.5 times more energy to raise than 1 calorie of protein from grains—incredible! That's not even counting how much rain forest is cut down to create grazing land for animals each year.

HERE'S ANOTHER WAY TO LOOK AT IT:
The Greenprint is the dietary version of a "carbon footprint"—the impact people and companies have on the environment, in terms of the greenhouse gases they have directly or indirectly caused, measured in units of carbon dioxide. CO_2 is a major polluter and dramatically harms our environment by adding to the greenhouse effect and causing global warming. The Greenprint measures how your food choices impact your health as well as clears away your carbon footprint.

By following a plant-based diet, you can reduce your carbon footprint by 1,560 kilograms of carbon dioxide equivalents annually. This is a bigger reduction than if you switched from driving a gas-guzzling SUV to a hybrid-electric Prius.

You can even make a huge impact with the most incremental changes in your diet. Even if you ate one less hamburger a week for one year, this would be the equivalent of driving 320 fewer miles.

So just think of the impact on the environment if everyone in the country cut their meat intake by half and made up the difference with wholesome plant foods, such as whole grains, legumes, vegetables, fruits, nuts, and seeds. That's why embracing meatless menus can mean a lot to our earth—even if it's not every meal or every day.

Healthwise, your greenprint has an extraordinary impact on your health. Let me give a rundown of just some of the health-building benefits of plant foods. Research has shown that plant-based eating, and this plan in particular:

// Takes off pounds rapidly and consistently, plus prevents overweight and obesity because plant foods make you feel fuller with fewer calories

// Fights diabetes. One in three Americans now has diabetes or prediabetes, and it's one of the leading causes of death.

// Keeps your heart healthy by lowering cardiovascular risk factors such as hypertension, clogged arteries, and abnormal clot formation

// Naturally detoxifies your body against cancer-causing agents

// Eases arthritis and joint pain

// Strengthens your immune system so that you rarely become ill

// Boosts your memory and wards off dementia

// Preserves your vision and protects your eyes from cataracts and macular degeneration

// Makes your skin, hair, and nails glow

That's the power of plants!

BIRTH OF A PLANT-BASED REVOLUTION

My greenprint is about what I eat, the choices I make, and how I conduct my life. As a father of four, I know that my choices now will affect my children's health and the earth they will inherit in the future.

The development of the Greenprint program is something that evolved from deep within my family history. I grew up in the '70s and have so many amazing memories of my youth. My mom raised my brother, sister, and me as a single parent, and we'd see our father every other week or so.

We spent a lot of time at my grandmother's house. Mima, as we called her, was so funny, and it wasn't even deliberate. She would say or do something on a daily basis that would immediately cause us to crack up. Then she'd look at us and ask why we were laughing (*"De que se ríen?"*), which would make us laugh even more.

My brother, Alfredo, whom I called Tito from an early age because I couldn't pronounce Alfredito (it's quite common in Spanish culture to add *-ito* to the end of a kid's name to make it more youthful), would love going over to Mima's house because he knew it would always be an adventure. I can still hear the ice cream truck driving by with its jingle playing over a loudspeaker. An almost orchestrated scream coming from the neighborhood kids would follow—*"El heladero!!!! El heladero!!!!"* ("The ice cream man!!! The ice cream man!!!")—and everyone would run outside with loose change, chasing the truck. Often, the driver would act like he didn't see us all running behind the truck. He would drive what felt like a few extra blocks (actually just a few extra feet), then he'd laugh along with us as we caught our breath and placed our orders. What amazing times.

Mima didn't drive, but she loved to get out. I can remember walking for hours every day as we visited all the shops, bodegas, and houses she would take us to.

It was nonstop at Mima's house. She'd make us a homemade lunch (usually something with chicken), and it was always delicious. Around lunchtime, she'd also always take all these tiny little pills. Mima suffered from heart problems. She used to tell me they were hereditary and that everyone in her family had them. Well, I assumed it was normal because she was old. I can remember that on occasion she'd get winded and would put a tiny little pill under her tongue, and a few minutes later she was much better. I later found out that those tiny little pills were nitroglycerin, which was for her angina, a chest pain caused by reduced blood flow to the heart.

Mima wasn't the only member of my family with health problems. Others were either sick or on some type of medication for hypertension, diabetes, or anxiety. Watching all this as a kid triggered my desire to study medicine. I can remember telling Mima, "When I grow up, I'm going to become a doctor and take care of you."

Fast-forward many years, and despite the medications, not much improved. It actually all worsened. My grandfather on my dad's side went blind due to his diabetes. My great-grandmother on my mom's side died of cancer. So did my maternal grandfather. My father died of heart failure. Mima suffered a stroke and was paralyzed as a result; she eventually passed away but lived in bed, immobile, for years.

Each one of these family members lived well into their eighties—my grandfather actually made it to ninety-six—but their quality of life was poor. And that was the tragedy to me—living in poor health is not really living.

I thought about this deep and hard. My father was on blood pressure medication from the time I was born, when he was in his thirties. Mima was only in her forties when I was born and was already taking medication she would continue to take for the rest of her life.

Why didn't someone tell them that changing the way they were eating could help? Why didn't they do anything to improve their lifestyle? Why? Didn't they care? Yes, they did—they just didn't have the right information to help them change.

I so desperately wanted to help Mima and my other family members regain their health. This desire stayed with me throughout high school. It was the number one reason I wanted to become a doctor. Ultimately, I chose not to attend medical school because I felt I could help more people through a preventative lifestyle rather than a reactive medical system. I wanted to touch lives and make sure people did not have to suffer a declining quality of life because of their poor choices and inherited habits.

As I studied nutrition, I learned about the power of plants, but I wanted to know even more. I kept reading, studying, researching, and talking to other plant-based advocates wherever I went. The more I learned, the more I leaned toward plant-based eating. Eventually I realized plant-based living was something I had to experience for myself. And that's exactly what I did. First, I gave up dairy. That felt so good that I stopped eating red meat and pork, then chicken and eggs. So far, so good. The last animal product to go was fish.

I did it gradually, but as time went on, I grew bolder. I became a vocal advocate of the plant-based lifestyle. "Eat plants" became my mantra.

What made me stick to this new lifestyle was knowing that I was, for the first time ever, truly in control of my health and impacting the planet in a positive way, while influencing others to do the same. This became the concept I eventually dubbed the Greenprint.

Many of my relatives lived long lives. But the Greenprint isn't just about living a longer life—it's about living a *better* life. A *fuller* life. A life where you can continue to enjoy yourself into your sixties, seventies, eighties, nineties, and beyond. Your best life. The life that my Mima deserved. The life we all deserve. The life our planet deserves.

But where do we start? What do we have to do to make a difference? How do we transform our lives and the planet with our personal greenprint?

INTRODUCING THE GREENPRINT

At its heart, the Greenprint is a program for a health transformation. It is also a blueprint for plant-based eating. And yes, it is vegan, but with a difference. A vegan diet is not necessarily plant-based. You can be a vegan and live on potato chips, pretzels, and vegan hot dogs served on gluten-free bread. But these processed foods can make you just as sick and unhealthy as a meat-inclusive diet, and they are not part of a plant-based diet. When I say "plant-based," I mean plants, not foods made in a plant. I'm talking about a diet that consists of 100 percent delicious foods that come from the earth. I'm talking about a diet that your body loves.

Ultimate success at plant-based living comes from a couple of factors that impact each other. If you want to flourish, if you want to enjoy your happiest life, there are two key components of the Greenprint: twenty-two laws of plant-based living, and the application of those laws in your life.

THE TWENTY-TWO
GREENPRINT LAWS

Whether we think so or not, it is part of human nature to search out a set of rules by which to live. And if you have never eaten 100 percent plant-based before, you will want to learn the most effective and most powerful rules to live by. In the case of the Greenprint, there are twenty-two. You can choose to ignore these laws, and possibly flirt with weight gain and health disasters, or you can learn them, adopt them, and mold your food choices and habits around them, and live an amazingly healthy life.

I developed these laws through clinically proven science and data, by living a completely plant-based lifestyle myself, and by helping others transition to plant-based eating. If I have learned anything over the past twenty-plus years, it is that what works in a clinical setting doesn't always work in the real world, which is why these laws are as practical as they are scientific.

A lot of people think they're doing "okay" with their nutrition choices. Others are flailing and failing. Still others are confused about what to eat or what diet to follow, because there are too many "flavor of the month" diets thrown at them. These diets are hyped, but there's little credibility behind the hype. Some people may want that secret potion, that magical weight-loss elixir, but it honestly doesn't exist. If you believe it does, you'll spend your life in a rabbit hole of diets, filled with empty promises that will most likely leave you weak, overweight, and sick.

The truth is, diets don't work simply because they are unrealistic and do not offer people the opportunity to develop a lifetime of healthful eating habits—"lifetime" being the operative word here. Diets are a quick fix for a long-term problem, which is often poor eating habits. A diet might work for a month or two, but most people drop the diet within a relatively short period.

Because of this mess, there's no clear standard, no boundaries, no real finish line on what to eat and what to avoid. People have forgotten how to make sound nutrition choices. This is why we need these twenty-two laws. In terms of nutrition, we live in a confusing world—how you emerge from that confusion will be determined by whether you implement the twenty-two distinct laws that I reveal to you in this book.

Learning the Greenprint laws gives you the essential knowledge you need to maintain your and your family's health. The laws crystallize your thinking and serve as a road map to success. In part 1 of this book, I lay out the twenty-two Greenprint laws. They are a prelude to action—a real master plan for a health-altering, energy-boosting, body-strengthening, and planet-saving lifestyle. Whether you are already eating a lot of plants or are more the "steak 24/7" type, implementing the Greenprint laws will be life-changing. Knowing and understanding them is the first step in my Greenprint program. If you choose to apply them, they can take you wherever you want to go.

> **THE GREENPRINT** *ISN'T JUST ABOUT LIVING A LONGER LIFE—IT'S ABOUT LIVING A BETTER LIFE.*

THE GREENPRINT DIET

In part 2, I'll show you how to put these laws into action, with a nutrition program that will help you start your journey in an achievable way that will yield powerful results: sustainable weight loss, more energy, and protection against life-shortening diseases.

The program is structured in three transitional tiers that allow you to progress at your own pace, experiment, and learn. I ask you to approach plant-based eating one meal at a time—just like I did in the beginning—until you eventually go 100 percent plant-based. I won't overwhelm you on the first day. I won't ask you for instant change. I won't tell you to throw out the way you eat overnight and go all or nothing with me—unless you want to! You have that option. Over the years, I have worked with thousands of people to successfully change their diets and their health, but what I realized on my own journey is that no single plan will work for everyone. An all-or-nothing proposition can be a recipe for failure, depending on your personality. That's where the Greenprint is different.

The Greenprint program shows you how to make small changes—the twenty-two most effective ones—to make a difference in your body, your health, and the planet. The program meets you where you are on your journey, and helps you improve your personal greenprint for the better, whittle your waistline, achieve superior health, and drain your carbon stream.

In Tier 1, you'll eat one plant-based meal a day for eleven days. In Tier 2, you'll enjoy two plant-based meals each day for eleven days. And in Tier 3—voilà!—you'll be ready to fully transition to 100 percent plant-based eating. Tier 3 includes a forty-four-day plan with specific, easy, and delicious meal suggestions, recipes, and tips for stocking your pantry.

This stepwise approach makes it easy to experiment with delicious meals, allowing you to incorporate the foods you love. By initially focusing on just one or two meals at a time, you'll gain the confidence to fully embrace plant-based eating for a lifetime. With the Greenprint, you'll take the time to get it right.

THE HOLY NAME STUDY
AND THE GREENPRINT

To put the Greenprint to the test, my team and I worked with Holy Name Medical Center, ranked one of the top hospitals in New Jersey by *U.S. News & World Report,* to study the benefits of plant-based eating on the body.

The study was born from a conversation between Holy Name Medical Center's Director of Cardiac Catheterization Dr. Angel Mulkay and President and CEO Michael Maron. Mr. Maron wanted to compare a vegan versus vegetarian lifestyle and the impact it could have on overall well-being and clinical markers. From there a study was developed and approved by the Institutional Review Board (IRB).

This trailblazing clinical trial measured the effects of three different diets over twenty-two days. More than 200 participants were recruited and randomized into one of three cohorts: 1. Western diet (animal-based); 2. vegetarian diet (dairy and plant-based); and 3. plant-based diet (no dairy or animal products). Each participant signed a consent form and kept a food diary.

In addition, the plant-based group received, at their homes, prepackaged vegan meals from my company for twenty-two days. The vegetarian group received meals prepared in-house for them by their food and nutrition department. The Western diet group simply followed a typical Western-type diet that included animal foods.

All participants had the following tests prior to and after the twenty-two-day test period:

// STYKU body scanning

This is a very high-tech scanning system that extracts waist, hip, bust, and hundreds of other body measurements and calculates them with less than 1 percent error. You simply stand on a turntable and hold still for 30 seconds while the platform spins. With its sharp high-resolution infrared images, this technology captures millions of data points in a matter of seconds in a fast, noninvasive process.

// Blood work

- Complete blood count (CBC)
- Lipid profile (including total cholesterol, LDL cholesterol, and triglycerides)
- B_{12} (for the vegan cohort)
- HgA1C (a blood sugar measurement that determines risk of diabetes)

After twenty-two days, the blood work results were astonishing when vegans versus vegetarians were compared:

// 5% decrease in BMI (a decrease greater than five times more than the vegetarians)

// 19% decrease in LDL (a decrease of 85% more than the vegetarians)

// 13% decrease in cholesterol (a decrease of over 400% more than the vegetarians)

// A decrease in body fat of over 400% more than vegetarians (as measured by STYKU)

// An average decrease in weight of 8 pounds lost (almost five times more weight loss than the vegetarians)

The participants in the vegan cohort reported:

// Feeling more energetic

// Improved skin and hair

// Better digestion

// Improved sleep quality, including needing less sleep

Two participants who suffered from migraines reported not having headaches while on the diet, and they no longer needed to take their preventive medication. Others reported decreased use or elimination of cholesterol and blood pressure medication.

The same can happen to you! Throughout this book, you'll meet several people who benefited from 100 percent plant-based eating. They did it easily, with amazing results, and they'll inspire you to do the same. In fact, after doing the Greenprint program, expect to:

// **LOSE WEIGHT**—up to a pound a day—as you focus entirely on plant-based foods and rid your body of preservatives and additives. Week by week, you will undoubtedly have more energy and feel lighter on the scale, while stamping your own greenprint on the global warming crisis. If you've tried to lose weight in the past, you may think it's as simple as taking in fewer calories than you burn. Yet not all calories are the same; the Greenprint proves this. When you eliminate meat, dairy, and processed foods from your diet, you also eliminate the primary sources of unhealthy fat and slash your caloric intake as well—without suffering from hunger pangs or sugar cravings.

// **ACCELERATE WEIGHT LOSS.** You will harness a strategy known as intermittent fasting, or going without food for specific amounts of time, typically overnight. Research has shown that intermittent fasting not only speeds weight loss but boosts metabolism, reduces inflammation, and improves cellular function while promoting longevity.

// **EXPERIENCE AMAZING, SATISFYING TASTES**—which is what makes this program so remarkable. You'll learn how to enjoy an astonishing array of vegetables, fruits, grains, and plant-based proteins. People have said to me, "I can't eat plant-based . . . I'm too much of a foodie." Well, guess what? I am a *huge* foodie. Trust me, food never tasted as good as the dishes you will discover here. Even a die-hard meat-and-potatoes person can make the switch without too much adjustment.

SAVE YOUR HEART. You no longer have to worry that you're eating a lot of artery-clogging saturated fat as you do when eating animal-based foods. Instead, by selecting healthy unsaturated fats—mainly from nuts, seeds, avocados, and other whole foods—you can lower your cholesterol and triglyceride levels.

DETOXIFY YOUR BODY NATURALLY. You will be consuming fewer pesticides, chemicals, hormones, and antibiotics, and eating more plant detoxifiers that help your body naturally cleanse itself around the clock.

REVERSE AGING AND REV UP YOUR HEALTH. You'll learn how embracing this lifestyle can help boost your energy; reduce inflammation; improve your overall health; help reduce the risk of, and even prevent, diseases like heart disease, cancer, and diabetes, the leading killers; and even extend your life expectancy. It doesn't hurt that top health experts are coming forward with scientific proof of the benefits of diets based on plants versus those based on animals. You'll discover that knowledge through this book.

And that's just scratching the surface!

While applying the twenty-two laws, you will significantly expand your greenprint. In fact, what makes this program unique is that you can use it not only as a guide to plant-based eating for optimal health and weight loss, but also as a road map to actively curbing carbon, reducing greenhouse gases, saving animals, and reducing global warming with your food choices. And you'll have the tools to figure out your personal greenprint.

The first step on the journey to successful plant-based living is a shift in your mind-set: Decide what's important to you, and what you want to accomplish. Do you want better health? A lower number on the scale? Sounder sleep? The knowledge that you've made a positive impact on the planet? Or maybe it's some combination of these. Whatever your reason, the kind of person you are begins and ends in your own mind. This isn't a new idea—it's been around since ancient times. You become what you think about most, so if you want to be healthier or lose weight or reduce your carbon footprint, you have to change the way you think.

Focus not on what you have to give up, but instead on all the good things you will gain—which can be summed up in one word: *life*. A happy one. A healthy one. One in which joy is spilling over.

The choice is yours.

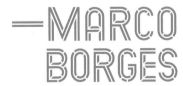

—MARCO BORGES

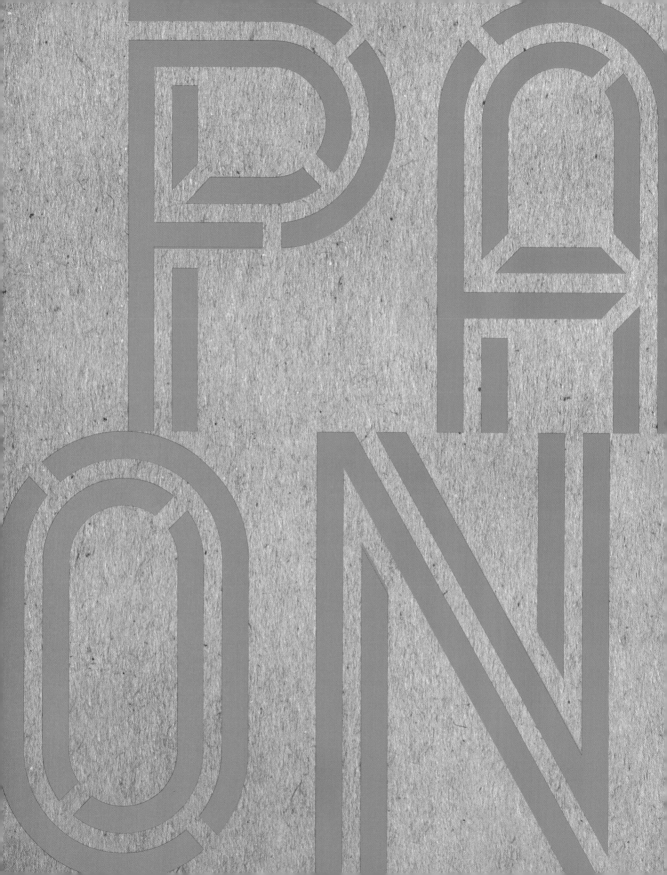

LAWS

//////

THE TWENTY-TWO GREENPRINT LAWS ////

break down what it takes to become successful in your transition to plant-based living. They give you standards to aspire to, while providing practical suggestions for developing a lifetime of healthier eating habits. I start with laws that address food choices that can create the state of health you want for yourself. Keep reading from there, and you'll discover more about how these laws can also help you become part of the solution to our global warming crisis.

THE LAWS ARE VITAL because they contain details that even the most health-conscious eaters have been missing—details that can save your health and are designed for long-term sustainable weight loss.

Every single law reveals critical steps to create lasting health success. My suggestion is to read the laws sequentially as they are presented, then reflect on each one. What resonates with you? What inspires you? What moves you to action?

The laws are also geared toward helping you form better habits. When I was growing up, I was curious about the behaviors that led to success in all realms of life. One question nagged at me: Why can some people completely turn their lives around while others struggle with the same problems again and again?

As I continued to observe people's behaviors, the answer became obvious: Making positive choices led to positive results. I saw the force of positive habits more and more through my work in the fitness industry. Most high achievers take care of themselves with exercise and good eating habits. Without good health, they can't achieve.

When it comes to habits, too often we put on emotional blinders. We refuse to look at ourselves objectively because we might not like what we see. But in order to change what you do, you must observe your habits objectively, without emotion. Why do you do the things you do? Why do you feel the way you feel? Why do you think what you think? The laws will help you become more self-aware so that you can figure out who you want to be, how you want to feel, and where you want to go with your health.

If you spend your energy worrying that shifting to a plant-based lifestyle will be hard, you'll stay stuck in your old ways. Our food is changing, and not for the better, and your health depends on your ability to adapt. The more you take this new lifestyle one step at a time, the more confident you'll become in your ability to adapt and create positive habits in your life.

The truth is that no matter who you are, how much money you have, whether you have five children or none, whether you are a man or a woman, whether you are young or old, you have habits—those little things you do every day, all the time, whether you are thinking about doing them or not. They are the actions that got you where you are and will keep you there in the future.

The laws are meant to help you forge positive habits—and make daily positive choices that will really affect you in the long run. So please, take the laws to heart. Follow the guidelines they propose to create the health you want. They can really make a difference if you follow them consistently.

In the end, following the laws will ensure that your future is better than your past.

EAT MORE PLANTS

AND LESS OF EVERYTHING ELSE

> People need to eat whole-food plant foods, primarily . . . whole grains, fruits, vegetables, nuts, and seeds. That diet supports our lives. We ought to live to be ninety or one hundred without getting any diseases.

—JOHN MACKEY,
cofounder of Whole Foods Market and
American business leader

YOU'VE HEARD IT YOUR ENTIRE LIFE: "Eat your vegetables." Whoever said it may not have known exactly why, but that didn't make them wrong. You know why? Plants are *life*! That's why this is Law #1. Allow me to remind you: Eat more vegetables, and eat *more* vegetables while you're at it.

Add fruits, beans, legumes, seeds, nuts, and whole grains, and the wide-ranging plant world can easily make up your *entire* diet. Plants offer us such an amazing array of foods that there's bound to be something even the biggest vegetable skeptic can love.

A plant-based diet can revitalize your body and your health in ways you may not think are possible. The results of the Holy Name study prove this: your LDL cholesterol can drop, perhaps by as much as 19 percent, as it did in the study. You'll lose inches from all over your body. Remember, the plant-based eaters in the study lost on average 8 pounds in just twenty-two days. They also reduced their blood pressure and improved their digestion, among other amazing improvements.

One of those plant-based eaters was Bridget, director of medical records at Holy Name Medical Center. She was happy that she had been randomly selected to be in the plant-based group of our study. She was not a vegan, though she's an avowed animal lover and concerned about the ethics of animal agriculture—so much so that she and her husband take in all sorts of animals, from rabbits to goats to sheep and any animal that has been abandoned. "Our goal is to give animals a good life," she explained, and Bridget and her husband accomplish this mission on their farm.

Bridget's results from participating in the twenty-two-day study were surprising. Patchy skin problems cleared up. Her hair began to shine. She dropped 7 pounds. She felt better and had more zip. "I never, ever felt hungry. I was always satisfied," she said. "Anything that pushes that shift to eat less animal products rather than more is good."

The proof is in the change in her vital measurements, which astonished Bridget. Prior to the study, her vitals were:

> *Triglycerides*: 125
>
> *Cholesterol*: 230
>
> *LDL*: 136
>
> *Weight*: 156
>
> *Body Mass Index (BMI)*: 30.4

After twenty-two days, take a look at what happened to Bridget:

> *Triglycerides*: 104
>
> *Cholesterol*: 219
>
> *LDL*: 122
>
> *Weight*: 149
>
> *BMI*: 29.1

"I've thought more about the food I eat than I ever have before, and I care about what I'm putting in my body," Bridget concluded.

To me, "Eat more plants" is a pretty simple law to follow. My family and I enjoy a 100 percent plant-based diet, which studies have found to be the only diet in the world that can prevent, arrest, and, in many cases, reverse heart disease. We also know that it's a cruelty-free way to live that is as good for the planet as it is for us. I have one simple guideline: I don't eat anything produced from or by something that has a face. This means no chicken, turkey, cows, pigs, sheep, or fish of any kind. This also means I don't eat dairy foods, including milk, cheese, or butter, and I don't eat eggs. I don't use mayonnaise or honey, either.

One of the questions I'm asked most frequently is, "What do you eat?" The answer is that I eat anything, as long as it doesn't originate from an animal. I eat vegetables, fruits, beans, legumes, grains, seeds, and nuts, and no, I never feel sluggish or weak, and I always get enough protein.

Of course, that's the big question you get when you stop eating meat: "How do you get enough protein?" Honestly, we are all eating more protein than we could ever need. We are not protein-deficient, and don't let anyone or any source tell you otherwise. There are plenty of studies that prove this beyond a shadow of a doubt. In fact, studies have shown that the more animal protein we eat, the sicker we will get.

The average daily requirement of protein is 46 grams for women and 56 grams for men. Scientists at Loma Linda University in California conducted the largest study in history of nutrient profiles of vegetarians, vegans, and non-vegetarians. It put to rest once and for all the perennial question, "Do vegetarians and vegans get enough protein?" The study followed more than seventy thousand adults for close to six years and calculated their intake of protein, along with other major nutrients such as vitamins and minerals.

According to this landmark study, non-vegetarians get way more protein than they need, and so does everyone else. On average, vegans and vegetarians get 70 percent more protein than they even require, and 97 percent of all Americans get enough protein.

So no one is really lacking protein. But there is another nutrient that 97 percent of Americans are deficient in: fiber. A fiber deficiency contributes to all sorts of life-threatening illnesses, from obesity to heart disease to diabetes to cancer. This nutrient is something we should be concerned about, not protein! (More on fiber in Law #3.)

We typically think of protein as coming from animal products. But the best sources of proteins are plant-based: beans, whole grains, nuts, and seeds. Even vegetables like spinach have protein. When you eat a well-rounded, varied, plant-based diet, you get all the protein you need.

So—let's stop obsessing over protein as the "cure" for obesity, overweight, diabetes, and other diseases. Let's start obsessing instead—in a positive way—about eating enough food that grows from the ground or in trees.

Plants top the diets that protect against heart disease, stroke, cancer, high blood pressure, cataracts, and macular degeneration. Cancer is often chalked up to bad genes. But according to Colin Campbell, professor emeritus at Cornell University and author of *The China Study*, "This is not about genes. Cancer is a function of nutrition." In fact, he has called the component of cow's milk known as casein "the most relevant chemical carcinogen ever identified." Another plant-based advocate, Dr. Caldwell Esselstyn, makes equally unequivocal statements about heart disease: "Heart disease need never exist. It is a food-borne illness."

Clearly, science and growing numbers of scientists support plant-based eating. Research shows that both high blood pressure and high blood sugar—risk factors for diabetes, cardiovascular disease, and stroke—begin to fall and normalize *within just a week* of starting a plant-based diet.

You don't need to eat animals to get nutrients besides protein, either. You can obtain all the carbohydrates, fats, vitamins, and minerals you need from plants, too.

Think about it: Where did the nutrition in the animals you have been eating come from? Plants! Plants are the original source of all nutrients. Nutrient-rich plant-based meals will make you leaner and, in the long run, healthier. You will feel great, with your body buzzing with energy and nutrition. Life will become so much easier. Developing the habit of eating plants gives you the energy, strength, and health to deal with life successfully—the energy to live your life in a positive, kind, and compassionate way, and to make the right choices for yourself, so you can be the healthiest version of yourself, inside and out. What are those choices? Take a look.

BEANS AND LEGUMES // When it comes to plant-based sources of protein, you can't go wrong with a few beans. Or lentils. One cup of cooked lentils can provide a whopping 18 grams of protein. Other great sources include black beans, kidney beans, and chickpeas, but truly, the options are endless when it comes to beans and legumes. Look for unique beans at your specialty foods store or the farmers' market. Eating beans or legumes in combination with grains is the easiest way to get all the essential amino acids—the vital tissue building blocks in protein—in one sitting.

GREEN VEGGIES // I am very pro-green vegetables. I eat a lot of them, because they are a source of all sorts of healthy vitamins and minerals, as well as fiber. If it's hard to find a place on your plate for plants, I say put them in your glass. Make a green smoothie every day. It takes five minutes, and tastes good, too. Even my children request them. Use whatever fresh fruit and veggies inspire you: spinach, kale, or chard, banana, berries, or pear. Add the liquid of your choice—I use water (no calories and nondairy), but you could try almond milk. The possibilities are endless—your smoothie will taste different every time but will always be nutritious.

COLORFUL VEGGIES // Vibrantly colored vegetables are more than just beautiful; they contain life-enriching phyto-chemicals. These chemicals provide flavor, color, scent, and valuable nutrients such as antioxidants and anti-inflammatories, which guard against many diseases, including diabetes, cancer, and heart disease. The more colors, the better.

THE PLANT-BASED DISTINCTION

Many people don't understand the differences among a vegetarian diet, a vegan diet, and a 100 percent plant-based diet.

VEGETARIAN

Eats milk and eggs, grains, and vegetables, but doesn't eat meat, poultry, or fish. There are variants of the vegetarian diet: ovo-lacto vegetarians eat eggs, dairy, and honey while excluding meat, fish, and poultry. Lacto-vegetarians exclude eggs, meat, fish, and poultry, but eat dairy and honey. Pesco-vegetarians eat fish, but not the flesh of other animals. And ovo-vegetarians eat eggs but exclude dairy from their diets.

VEGAN

Doesn't eat meat, poultry, fish, milk, eggs, or honey. Eats grains, vegetables, fruit, and, often, overprocessed vegan foods.

PLANT-BASED

Eats 100 percent plants—grains, vegetables, and fruits. Doesn't eat meat, poultry, fish, milk, eggs, honey, or processed vegan foods.

FRUIT // Eating just a small amount of fruit daily can reduce heart disease risk and improve health. According to an article published in the *New England Journal of Medicine* in 2016, researchers in China followed more than half a million people for seven years. They found that about 3.5 ounces (about 1 cup) of fresh fruit daily was enough to lower risk of heart attack and stroke. Apples, peaches, pears, berries, and other fruits all contain valuable heart-protective nutrients.

NUTS AND SEEDS // Both are terrific protein sources. Just ¼ cup of almonds contains 8 grams of protein, while 2 tablespoons of almond butter contain 7 grams. Pecans, walnuts, pistachios, and cashews are also great choices. When it comes to seeds, look for sunflower, pumpkin, hemp, chia seeds, and flaxseeds. Full of healthy fats and protein, these make great snacks, as well as additions to salads and side dishes. Be sure to keep an eye on your serving size of nuts and seeds, however, as they do pack a lot of calories.

WHOLE GRAINS // The latest USDA Dietary Guidelines for Americans noted that most people eat enough grains, but not enough *whole* grains. The whole grain has the most bang for the bite, including higher nutritional value and more flavor. Nutrients vary by grain type, but generally whole grains are rich in fiber, iron, potassium, magnesium, calcium, and B and E vitamins. A 2016 study in the journal *Circulation* reported that at least three servings of whole grains daily was associated with a 20 percent lower risk of death from all causes, and a 25 percent lower risk of death from cardiovascular disease. My favorites are whole-grain brown rice, quinoa, and steel-cut oats.

Quinoa (often classified and thought of as a grain, but actually a seed), in particular, is a great option and also lets you bump up your protein intake. One cup of cooked quinoa contains 8 grams of complete protein (containing all the essential amino acids), and if you combine it with other protein-rich foods, you'll quickly reach your recommended daily protein intake while also providing your body with lots of essential nutrients.

VEGAN PROTEIN POWDER // For a quick protein pick-me-up, you can't go wrong with a good plant-based protein powder. Have it in a smoothie as a quick and healthy breakfast or afternoon boost. You can even combine protein powder with some of your favorite recipes like brownies, muffins, and pancakes to ensure your meals are protein-packed. Look for USDA-certified organic protein powders with clean and simple ingredient profiles.

PLANT FATS // Be sure to eat delicious plant-based fats such as nut butters and avocados. Good fats slow the absorption of carbohydrates, help prevent disease, and provide important nutrients. Fats also help you feel full longer. They're great for energy, and you can add a tablespoon or two of them to your green smoothies.

EAT LESS JUNK

Let's pause here to consider the second part of this law: Eat less of everything else.

"And what is 'everything else'?" I hear you asking. Well, for one thing, it's junk food, and I'm sure you know exactly what that is: It's foods with questionable nutritional value laced with sugar and salt. It's soft drinks and other sugary beverages. It's highly processed, packaged food engineered with lab-produced flavors designed to be irresistible. It's the fast food sold on every corner of every town. You know it when you see it. When you do, don't eat it.

A lot of junk is filled with additives and artificial flavors, too. They trick your taste buds so much that they get confused when you eat real food because you're so used to chemicals. But when you remove artificially flavored foods from your diet, something magical happens. After a few days, your taste buds begin to function as they should. Suddenly you experience what an orange or carrot really tastes like. Or an apple, or a mango. You rediscover what sweet is really supposed to taste like.

Also under the heading of "everything else" are animal-based foods, such as meat and cheese. That massive study I mentioned on page 32 also compared the diets of those in the study who eventually died and those who did not. Vegetarians and vegans had a lower risk of death than non-vegetarians. The point is that eating too much animal-based food just might cut your life short. Why risk that?

When you follow this law, you will enjoy powerful results. As your new eating habits start to settle in, you will feel better and better—and learn that you actually love eating more fruits and vegetables on a regular basis. In fact, you will feel amazing, and you will begin to crave fresh, delicious plant foods.

You will notice this difference almost immediately. You will feel better and be healthier, and this will make you happier. Your amazing energy will come from those plants. When plants grow, the sun shines, energy is absorbed from the air and through the soil, and nature's chemistry turns light into food that gives you energy—pure, natural, healing energy that will change the way you live in the world.

YOUR GREENPRINT
by Following Law #1

You will become thinner, live longer, and be healthier—a point established by our Holy Name study, as well as the USDA's Dietary Guidelines, which state that vegetarian eating patterns, including vegan diets, may boost health by preventing obesity, slashing the risk of cardiovascular disease, and lowering total mortality.

NOBODY EVER PLANS TO FAIL

PEOPLE JUST FAIL TO PLAN

> Success
> depends upon
> previous
> preparation.
> —CONFUCIUS

WHEN YOU'RE SWITCHING TO PLANT-BASED EATING, planning is the key for success—and enjoyment! Set yourself up for success by anticipating your nutritional needs and making healthy, plant-based food accessible and convenient. Selecting healthy, life-giving foods for each of your three meals a day is possible—but just like any lasting change to your diet, it requires planning. It requires effort. Cucumbers don't buy themselves!

Some people bounce around from diet to diet, shedding pounds but then gaining it all back. It's frustrating. It's disheartening. If you want to stop failing, step out of the cycle of weight gain and disease and create a new cycle of vitality, planning and following through are the only way to get there. If you are looking for a get-thin-quick plan, you're in the wrong place. If you're looking for sustainable habits that will result in weight loss and great health, you're in the right place, because you are beginning an incredible journey toward optimum health and wellness. You're going to see what it feels like to take care of yourself and move toward being the best version of you.

The first step to changing the trajectory of your diet, weight, and health is to be completely accountable for where you are today—good or bad. Your parents aren't to blame, and neither is the economy or your favorite fast-food restaurant—you are. You are 100 percent responsible for everything you do; you will never fix your problems by blaming someone or something else. You choose what to eat, how to act, where to go, when to exercise (or not), and what foods to avoid.

Once you get all that straight, then you can get to the heart of how to plan for plant-based eating. When you plan, you win; when you don't, you fail.

PLANNING TO MEET YOUR NUTRIENT NEEDS

Reminder: Plant foods provide everything you need nutritionally. But ensuring that you receive all that "everything" requires thoughtful planning. Plan your meals around a variety of high-quality, nutrient-rich foods, such as whole grains, beans, legumes, vegetables, fruits, nuts, and seeds.

Plant-based eaters have to be a little more vigilant than most to get sufficient amounts of certain vitamins, minerals, and fats in their diets. The important nutrient targets to hit include:

IRON // One of the most common yet erroneous arguments against a plant-based diet is that it doesn't provide enough iron. In fact, those eating a meat-free, plant-based diet not only tend to get more iron, but also get more fiber, vitamins, and minerals. Plant-based iron, also known as non-heme iron, isn't absorbed as well as heme iron (which is found in animal blood and muscle) in the body, but studies show that avoiding heme iron has been associated with a reduced risk of heart disease, diabetes, stroke, and other chronic diseases.

A plant-based diet should include foods that are rich in iron, like kidney beans, black beans, soybeans, spinach, raisins (which are slightly higher in iron than grapes), cashews, oats, cabbage, and tomato juice (which has more iron than tomatoes).

Women require 18 milligrams of iron daily; men require 8 milligrams. For post-menopausal women, that drops to the same amount as for men, 8 milligrams. Pregnant women require 27 milligrams. Getting enough iron daily isn't difficult when you combine plant-based iron sources: A meal consisting of a cup of cooked spinach, a cup of quinoa, and half a cup of chickpeas contains about 12 milligrams of iron. A simple salad of spinach, dried currants, almonds, pumpkin seeds, and a few sun-dried tomatoes can easily deliver 10 milligrams of iron.

VITAMIN B$_{12}$ // Vitamin B$_{12}$ is abundant in meat, eggs, and dairy foods, and vegan diets get criticized because they don't supply enough of this nutrient. But one thing most people don't realize is that there's not even that much B$_{12}$ in beef anymore, because cows don't eat that much natural grass (the original source of this vitamin from bacteria that live in the soil). They are being injected with B$_{12}$!

The recommended daily amount of vitamin B$_{12}$ for adults is 2.4 micrograms, and you can get ample amounts from certain plant-based foods. Tempeh and miso, for example, contain high levels of this nutrient because it is produced by bacteria during fermentation. You can also obtain B$_{12}$ from nutritional yeast (a great condiment that tastes like Parmesan cheese), and some plant-based foods and cereals are fortified with it. Be careful that you get ample amounts of this

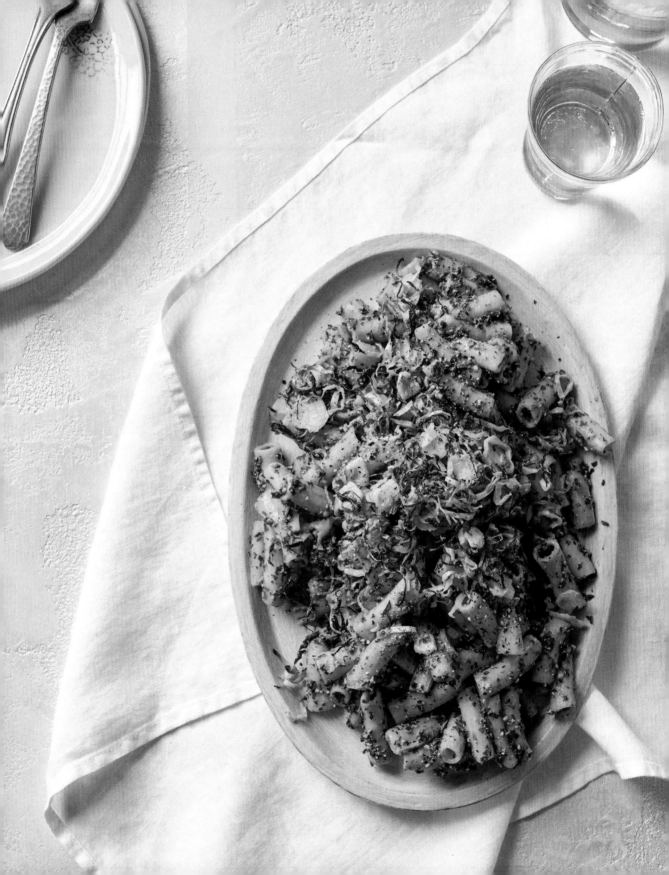

nutrient, as a B_{12} deficiency can be serious and even lead to irreversible nerve damage. I personally like to take a daily B_{12} supplement, which ensures that I'm getting exactly what I need. In our Holy Name study, the researchers had everyone in the vegan group take a B_{12} supplement. The participants levels of this important nutrient stayed normal, and, in some cases, even increased.

OMEGA-3 FATTY ACIDS // Although there is no official recommended daily allowance of omega-3 fatty acids, these fats play an important role in preventing chronic inflammation. They help form prostaglandins, a class of lipids that increase and decrease various functions relating to the inflammatory response, normal blood clotting, and the relaxation of blood vessels. Dietary sources of omega-3 fatty acids include flaxseeds and flax oil, soybeans and soybean oil, pumpkin seeds and pumpkin seed oil, tofu, walnuts and walnut oil, seaweed, and edible marine algae.

VITAMIN D // Vitamin D has been shown to reduce the risk of certain cancers and depression. It builds healthy bones and teeth, regulates insulin, and supports lung function and cardiovascular health.

Vitamin D intake is recommended at 400 to 800 IUs a day, or 10 to 20 micrograms. If you get fifteen minutes of sunlight each day, your body can produce ample vitamin D. Eating mushrooms is another way to obtain this vital nutrient.

CALCIUM // Dairy isn't the only source of this bone-building mineral, so don't fall for the rhetoric that vegans don't get enough calcium. All it takes is some planning and knowledge about the plant sources

of calcium, and you can easily reach the recommended daily amount.

The recommended daily amount for calcium is 1,000 milligrams for adults and children aged four years and older. A salad of two cups of kale, almonds, sunflower seeds, and white beans topped with a tahini dressing can total up to 500 milligrams of calcium. A smoothie made with a cup of nondairy milk (almond or other fortified nut milk), almond butter, and spinach will net you another 500 milligrams—more than meeting your daily requirements. Mustard and turnip greens, broccoli, collard greens, bok choy, and kale are also great calcium-rich foods. Consider, too, that while a cup of whole milk contains 288 milligrams of calcium, a quarter cup of sesame seeds provides 580 milligrams of calcium—nearly double that of milk. Sesame seed butter (known as tahini) is high in calcium and can be a delicious, rich-tasting addition to salads, hummus, vegetable dishes, and sandwiches.

PROTEIN // All plant foods contain protein. As I mentioned earlier, beans and legumes (including peas and lentils) are very popular plant-based sources of protein. One cup of cooked beans has the same amount of protein as 2 ounces of meat. Nuts and seeds are also full of protein.

ZINC // This four-letter trace element protects against infections and helps the body repair wounds. It's essential for growth and brain development in infants and children. The recommended daily amount for zinc is 15 milligrams for adults and children age four and older. You can meet this daily requirement easily by eating plenty of whole grains, legumes, and nuts.

PLANNING YOUR MEALS

How hard would it be to obtain all these nutrients? Well, the easiest way to find out (besides giving it a try) is to check out a typical day in the life of a plant-based eater. You'll see just how easy it is to cut out animal products and still get the nutrients your body needs.

BREAKFAST:
A HEALTHY SMOOTHIE

While on the weekends you might want to whip up something a bit fancier, for busy mornings, there's nothing better than a healthy, protein-packed, plant-based smoothie. Make your own with one cup of water (or nondairy milk), a banana, frozen berries, greens, flax/chia/hemp seeds, and a scoop of vegan protein powder. You'll start the day with lots of nutrients and be ready to hit the ground running. Alternatively, you can move your smoothie to the afternoon to head off the munchies and have a healthy bowl of oatmeal with fruit for breakfast instead.

LUNCH:
SUPER SOUPS AND SALADS

You can switch between soups and salads at lunch, or do both! Remember to include hearty fillings in your salad—black beans, quinoa, nuts, seeds, and so forth—in addition to any greens to keep your stomach full. Alternatively, throw the same salad ingredients in a gluten-free tortilla, and you have a wrap! The options for soups are endless, but you'll find that the best recipes have a good base, such as pureed sweet potato, cauliflower, or broccoli.

SNACKS AND SIDES

What works for you as a snack depends on whether you like sweet or salty. If you try to stick to healthy options, you'll notice you have more energy throughout the day. Snacks like fruits and veggies combined with nut or seed butters or hummus are terrific options.

DINNER:
THE MAIN EVENT

A plant-based lifestyle doesn't mean giving up good food! Soups, stews, casseroles, pizzas, burgers—it's all on the menu! A typical plant-based dinner would include a good source of protein, such as beans, legumes, or lentils, but could also use quinoa, artichokes, nuts or seeds, spinach, and so forth. It's easy to throw together a quick, healthy, plant-based meal of red kidney beans, quinoa, and broccoli, and top it with a cashew cream sauce. Delicious!

YOUR GREENPRINT
by Following Law #2

A well-planned plant-based diet supplies your body with more fiber, folic acid, vitamins C and E, potassium, magnesium, and many phytochemicals and contains less saturated fat than diets that contain animal products, as reported by a 2009 study in the *American Journal of Clinical Nutrition*.

EAT MORE, WEIGH LESS

> I've been on a constant diet for the last two decades. I've lost a total of 789 pounds. By all accounts, I should be hanging from a charm bracelet.
>
> —ERMA BOMBECK

FIGHTING FAT HAS BECOME A NATIONAL OBSESSION, but winning is often a lifelong battle, with major and minor victories along the way. Just ask rapper and songwriter Todd Gaither, who goes by the name Sauce Money. He is a veteran of the hip-hop industry, and for most of his life and career he was in a losing battle with his weight. At one point, he shot up to 500 pounds, which gave him painful and near-crippling stage 3 osteoporosis in his knees. He couldn't stand for longer than three minutes at a time. He had self-image problems in a business that can often be cruel if someone is overweight or obese.

"I sank into a dark place—something I wouldn't wish on anyone—because I was so obese. It was certainly no secret how big I was!" Sauce said. "People in my industry were dying all around me, and I knew I had to address my weight. I reached out to Jay-Z, a good friend of mine—we

> **"** **PLANT-BASED EATING** *IS THE MOST POWERFUL, MOST EFFECTIVE, AND EASIEST WAY TO LOSE WEIGHT—AND KEEP IT OFF.*

grew up together—for help. Jay-Z had gone vegan, and he put me in touch with Marco."

I worked very closely with Sauce, teaching him how to eat clean, plant-based foods. I knew he could do it because of his rise to prominence in the music world. I began seeing him as a lean, energetic guy and musician—someone proud of how he looked. I immediately put him on my eating plan. As with any lifestyle change, it was tough at first, but Sauce persevered—a mental discipline he learned in his college fraternity.

Sauce kept his diet simple: lots of beans, quinoa, and salads. Sure, there were a few bumps in the road, but he stuck to it like a champ. Over about two-and-a-half years, Sauce lost 200 pounds, and kept it off through his vegan lifestyle and working out five to six times a week with swimming, high-intensity cardio, and weight training. He no longer has any pain in his knees. He can now stand and continue to work very long

hours. Let me add that the very first change he noticed—and it happened in a matter of days—was that his complexion cleared up dramatically and he was super energetic for the first time in a long time.

Sauce told me that going plant-based was "the best thing I have ever done."

Sauce made his health a main priority. And now he believes if he can drop pounds, you can, too. In my most recent conversation with him, the rap star offered these words of encouragement:

"Simplify your diet. Begin by eating clean, whole foods: fresh fruits, vegetables, whole grains, and beans. Do the best you can.

"Become positively addicted to how great you feel. The longer you stay on a plant-based diet, the better you'll feel. It's like a wonder drug. You won't want to go back to your old ways. You can't 'unknow' what you now know and feel. Keep going forward; the future is full of possibilities.

"Get support from people who will never give up on you. For me, that was Jay-Z and Marco. They took the time to educate me. I owe them my life.

"Change your mind-set: You have to want to live longer and better than eat bad."

I couldn't have said it better myself, Sauce! As he discovered, by following a plant-based diet, you will control your weight, satisfy your hunger, and feel comfortably full after every meal. In fact, you can eat more to lose weight!

I know this law sounds like a dream come true if you've been shackled to restrictive diets that leave you feeling ravenous. Even though "eat less" is the mantra of the weight-loss industry, slimming down does not have to be about deprivation and hunger.

Plant-based eating is the most powerful, most effective, and easiest way to lose weight—and keep it off. And there's plenty of proof.

Following a plant-based diet fights fat around the waistline, for example. After tracking nearly eighty thousand healthy adults for ten years, American Cancer Society researchers found that men and women who ate nineteen or more servings of vegetables a week did not develop abdominal obesity—that is, they didn't get muffin tops or love handles—while those who ate meat more than seven times a week did! Gaining fat around the waist, or developing what's known as an "apple" shape, has been linked to heart disease, diabetes, and certain cancers.

This isn't the only study showing the power of plants as fat fighters. In a study conducted at the University of South Carolina and reported on the website of the Vegetarian Resource Group, fifty overweight adults were randomly assigned to one of five diets: a non-vegetarian diet, a semi-vegetarian diet (red meat once a week, poultry no more than five times a week), a pesco-vegetarian diet, a lacto-ovo vegetarian diet, or a vegan diet. They followed their assigned diet for two months and were not required to limit their caloric intake. After the initial trial, researchers encouraged the dieters to stick to their assigned diet for another four months.

All the dieters lost weight, but the vegan group lost the most—exactly what we found in our Holy Name study. After six months, the vegan eaters had shed an average of 7.5 percent of their starting weight. The way I see it, the exciting results of this study and others like it offer proof that a plant-based diet is an effective way to lose weight. I love all this great scientific evidence, but I'm not surprised. When clients come to me, most of them want to get slimmer and fitter. The first thing I do is show them how to incorporate more plants into their diets—and hopefully get them to go plant-based for life. At the same time, I encourage them to cut out the overprocessed foods that are slowly poisoning their bodies. Once they get on a true plant-based diet, I see them drop anywhere from 10 to 100 pounds (or more), as their excess fat melts away and they catapult themselves into a world of energy and vitality. All along, they are eating more food than ever before. They are not hungry, and they are shedding excess weight. Many people can lose up to a pound a day eating plants! Of course, as they're knocking off the pounds, they are simultaneously reversing and preventing lifestyle diseases.

A few years ago, I bumped into a friend at my kids' school. He casually mentioned that he had some friends who had switched to a plant-based diet following my dietary protocols, and that the results were amazing. I interpreted his remarks to be code for "I want to try it." At the time, he was tipping the scales at 300 pounds, on a six-feet-five frame.

I thanked him for his kind words and said that I'd be happy to guide him along the way if he was willing to give it a try. That very day, he was ready to jump in. He had one reservation, however: "I'm Cuban, like you are, and I love Cuban foods." I reminded him that a lot of Cuban food is plant-based: black beans, rice, corn, yuca, potatoes, tomatoes, lettuce, cucumbers, and plantains. In fact, the original Cuban diet was mostly vegetarian until the Spaniards, who ruled Cuba until the turn of the century, imported beef and pork and put meat into the cuisine. My friend was sold.

After a full day of eating plant-based, he called me.

"Bro, you do know that I'm trying to lose weight, right?"

"Yes, I know, why?"

"Dude, if I eat all the food you recommended, I'm definitely going to gain weight." I started to laugh, then explained to him that plant foods are much denser in nutrients but lighter in calories—the essence of Law #2. For example, a 16-ounce bag of spinach may be around 100 calories, while 16 ounces of animal protein might be ten times that (around 1,000 calories) with zero fiber! You'll wind up eating more but taking in fewer calories and getting a lot more fiber.

My friend sighed loudly. "I get to eat, I won't be hungry, and I'm going to lose weight? I'm all in."

Only a few months later, he had dropped more than 80 pounds, without feeling hungry at all.

Plain and simple: Plant-based eating gets results for every person I have ever worked with.

Why? What's the secret?

Well, one of the big secrets is fiber.

Fiber is funny stuff. We eat it, but we can't digest it, so it passes through the digestive tract, doing a bunch of amazing things for weight control and overall health along the way. As I mentioned earlier, 97 percent of Americans are deficient in fiber. In fact, we are so deficient in fiber that it has been listed as a nutrient of concern in the USDA's Dietary Guidelines. That's a problem we really need to work on!

FIBER AND YOUR HEALTH

Fiber is a health saver! It appears to reduce the risk of many illnesses:

ACNE AND RASHES. Fiber may help usher yeasts and fungi from your body, preventing them from being eliminated through your skin, where they could trigger acne or rashes.

BOWEL DISEASES. Fiber may ease irritable bowel syndrome (IBS) and other inflammatory conditions in the bowel.

BRAIN HEALTH. Fiber improves mood, cognition, and alertness.

CARDIOVASCULAR DISEASE. There is evidence that fiber helps prevent heart attacks, and research shows that people who eat a high-fiber diet have a 40 percent lower risk of heart disease.

CHRONIC INFLAMMATION. Dietary fiber appears to be anti-inflammatory, decreasing inflammation-associated markers, including C-reactive protein (CRP).

COLON CANCER. Fiber whisks toxins and cancer-causing agents from your digestive tract, which helps prevent cancer.

DIVERTICULAR DISEASE. Fiber (especially insoluble fiber) may reduce your risk of diverticulitis—an inflammation of the colon—by 40 percent.

GALLSTONES. A high-fiber diet may reduce the risk of gallstones because of fiber's ability to help regulate blood sugar.

HEMORRHOIDS. A high-fiber diet may lower your risk of hemorrhoids, which can be painful and cause blockages and bleeding.

INFECTIONS. Fiber improves the population of healthy bacteria in your gut—which means it can help prevent infections, including colds and flu.

INSULIN RESISTANCE. Fiber makes your cells more receptive to insulin. Insulin can thus do a better job of getting glucose into cells for energy.

KIDNEY STONES. A high-fiber diet may reduce the risk of kidney stones, likely because of its ability to help regulate blood sugar.

OBESITY AND OVERWEIGHT. Fiber has been shown to enhance weight loss among obese and overweight people, likely because it increases feelings of fullness.

STROKE. Researchers have found that for every 7 grams more fiber you consume on a daily basis, your risk of stroke decreases by 7 percent.

TYPE 2 DIABETES. Soluble fiber may help to slow the breakdown of carbohydrates and the absorption of sugar in the body, helping to control blood sugar.

HERE'S THE IMPORTANT POINT FOR ALL OF US: Eat more fiber from plant foods to enjoy all of its amazing health benefits.

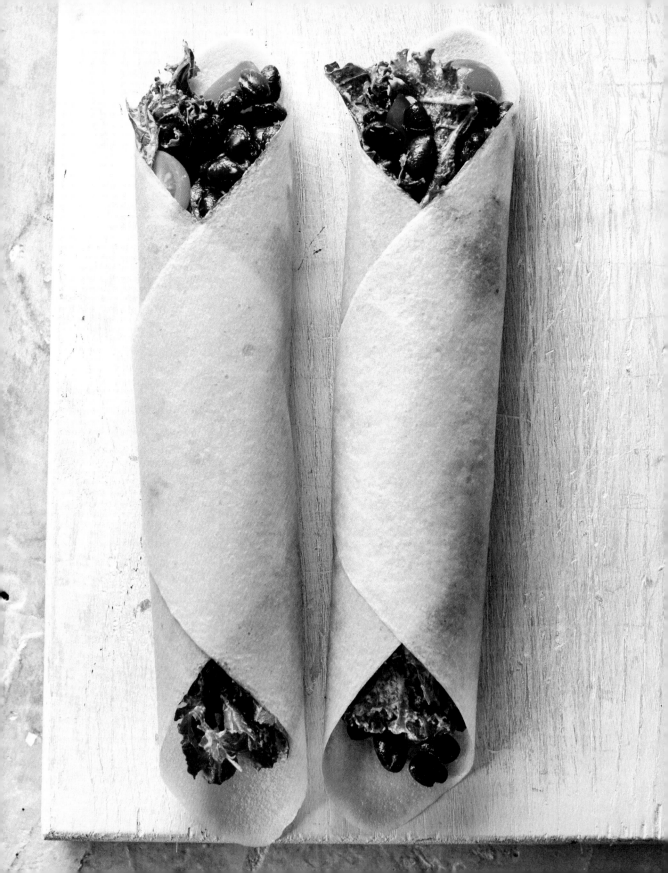

WHERE'S THE FIBER?

By definition, fiber is found only in plant foods, and nowhere else. But one of the problems behind our collective fiber deficiency is that most people have no idea what is in their food. In fact, more than half of Americans think steak is a source of fiber.

There are two categories of fiber: soluble and insoluble. Soluble fiber acts like a sponge; it soaks up excess cholesterol, fats, and toxins. Insoluble fiber is like a scrub brush; it "scours" the digestive tract as it passes through. We need both the sponge and the scrub brush to keep our systems clean.

Foods high in soluble fiber include oats and oat bran, barley, beans and legumes, apples, pears, and citrus fruits (but not fruit juices). Insoluble fiber is found mostly in the skins and husks of plant foods, whereas soluble fiber dwells in the fleshy part inside the fruit. For instance, apple peels are largely insoluble fiber, while the flesh of an apple is mostly soluble fiber.

Both categories of fiber do four powerful things to promote weight loss: **NUMBER 1:** Fiber tames your appetite so you don't overeat. There's a powerful hormone in your body called cholecystokinin (CCK) that helps control satiety, the feeling of fullness that stops hunger. Fiber increases the production and prolongs the activity of CCK. As a result, you'll feel fuller longer, and your cravings for fattening stuff will diminish. **NUMBER 2:** Fiber helps prevent the absorption of excess calories from the fat you eat. Because the body can't break down fiber, fiber exits the body in the same form it entered. As it moves through your body, it snatches up fat and whisks it all the way through to your colon, where the fat and fiber are packaged together into stool and eliminated from the body.

In a study by the USDA, researchers set a certain limit on calories for volunteers and altered the fiber content in their diets. They found that fewer calories were absorbed with increased fiber intake. People who took in up to 36 grams of fiber a day absorbed 130 fewer calories daily—automatically. Over a year, that adds up to around 47,000 calories. Because each pound of body fat is equal to 3,500 calories, you could lose nearly 14 pounds in a year—effortlessly—by increasing your daily fiber intake. **NUMBER 3:** Fiber slows down the conversion of carbohydrates to glucose (blood sugar) in your body. This helps prevent weight gain, because excess glucose not used for energy converts to triglycerides that are either stored as unwanted body fat or accumulate in the blood, where they cause artery-clogging plaque. Fiber also increases insulin sensitivity, which means that cells respond well to insulin when it brings glucose to their doors (receptors) as fuel. Over time, eating more fiber will help your body use glucose more efficiently; in other words, your body will become more of a natural "fat-burning" machine. **NUMBER 4:** Fiber helps populate the levels of beneficial bugs (probiotics) in your gut—a factor that can improve your shape. Your body hosts trillions of these tiny critters, most of whom hang out in your intestines. They break down food, help you absorb certain nutrients, and keep your immune system running at peak efficiency.

But here's the hitch: There's now surprising evidence that the wrong gut bugs may make you prone to put on weight. In one study, researchers discovered that a virus called adenovirus-36 (Ad-36)—a bug known to make chickens fatter—was three times more prevalent in the guts of obese people than in the guts of lean people. Also, some gut bacteria trigger cravings and a tendency to store more calories as fat.

Happily, the trick is to make sure the good bugs outnumber the bad. One important way to do this is to feed the good bugs their favorite food: special prebiotic fibers found in a variety of plant foods, like asparagus, Jerusalem artichokes, onions, garlic, and leeks, as well as chia seeds, flaxseeds, and hemp seeds. Nurturing the beneficial creatures in your digestive tract may be a helpful route to a healthy weight.

Of course, there's almost no end to the number of trendy diets you can participate in. But thanks to these four factors, the safest and most natural way to shed pounds is simply to eat a fiber-rich plant-based diet. They make fiber a fantastic secret weapon in the fight against fat! I'll show you how to apply this wellness law to your life in part 2, but let's talk about how to start incorporating it now. For starters, how much fiber do you need each day to shed pounds, keep your weight under control, and stay healthy? The current medical recommendation is up to 35 grams, but no fewer than 25 grams,

of fiber daily. Sadly, most adults get only 15 grams or less!

You could hit (and exceed) that target by eating these foods over the course of a day: half a cup of oatmeal (3 grams fiber), one cup of raspberries (8 grams), half a cup of cooked red or black beans (7 grams), a small apple (5 grams), half a cup of cooked lentils (8 grams), and one cup of cooked peas (8 grams). That's 39 grams of fiber.

There are other simple actions you can take to automatically get into the high-fiber habit:

// Have 1/2 to 1 cup of oats or whole-grain cereal for breakfast.

// Sprinkle your cereal with chia seeds or flaxseeds.

// Toss a couple of handfuls of greens such as spinach into your smoothies.

// Snack on fresh fruit or nuts and seeds.

// Use avocado on toast and sandwiches, and in salads and smoothies (1/2 avocado contains 5 grams of fiber).

// Bake with high-fiber flours. For example, 1 ounce of coconut flour has 11 grams of fiber, and the same amount of soy flour has 5 grams of fiber.

// Chow down on plenty of beans and legumes, an important part of many traditional diets. Just one cup of cooked beans can deliver up to 75 percent of your daily fiber needs. Incorporate these fiber-rich foods into your diet by enjoying hummus and other bean dips or by topping salads with cooked beans or lentils.

// Eat plenty of green leafy vegetables, as well as vegetables with high water content such as cucumbers and tomatoes. You end up with a larger portion of fiber and water, which will fill you up before you get too many calories.

// Add a bean soup or salad to your dinner to help you feel more satisfied.

A lot of people have asked me why I eat a high-fiber and plant-based diet, since I am naturally thin and don't need to lose weight. It's true—I've never had a weight problem. But here's the beauty of it all: Not only will this law help you control your weight, but a high-fiber diet also resolves constipation and other digestive problems. The other advantages are that it can reduce the risk of heart disease, diabetes, high blood pressure, and some types of cancer. Preventing these illnesses is important to me, because there is a history of heart disease in my family. Eating a plant-based diet high in fiber makes me feel like I am ensuring myself against future problems.

As this law states, a high-fiber, plant-based diet lets you eat more food yet weigh less. It's satisfying enough to enjoy on an ongoing basis. While most diets are notoriously difficult to stick with, this law sets forth diet principles you can live with for a lifetime.

YOUR GREENPRINT
by Following Law #3

Transitioning to plant-based eating keeps you naturally thinner. Consider the following data: Vegetarians are significantly slimmer than meat eaters. On average, vegetarian men weigh nearly 17 pounds less than non-vegetarians, according to an analysis of multiple studies by researchers at Loma Linda University in California. And vegans are the slimmest of all, according to a British study of thirty-eight thousand meat eaters, fish eaters, vegetarians, and vegans, published in June 2003 in the *International Journal of Obesity*.

TOP 5 HIGH-FIBER FOODS

IN PLANT-BASED FOOD GROUPS

PLANT PROTEINS	SERVING SIZE	TOTAL FIBER (GRAMS)
The plant protein food group includes a variety of high-fiber items, which are also good sources of iron, zinc, and other vitamins and minerals. Try to have ½ to 1 serving of a plant protein at each meal.		
Lentils, cooked	1 cup	15.6
Black beans, cooked	1 cup	15.0
Lima beans, cooked	1 cup	13.2
Almonds	1 ounce (23 nuts)	3.5
Pistachio nuts	1 ounce (49 nuts)	2.9

VEGETABLES	SERVING SIZE	TOTAL FIBER (GRAMS)
The vegetable group includes both raw and cooked vegetables. This group is especially high in disease-fighting antioxidants and life-enriching phytochemicals. Eat liberally from this group.		
Artichoke, cooked	1 medium	10.3
Green peas, cooked	1 cup	8.8
Broccoli, cooked	1 cup	5.1
Turnip greens, cooked	1 cup	5.0
Brussels sprouts, cooked	1 cup	4.1

FRUITS	SERVING SIZE	TOTAL FIBER (GRAMS)
The fruit group includes raw fresh fruit. Eating just a small amount of fruit daily can reduce heart disease risk and improve your health. Enjoy 1 to 2 servings daily.		
Raspberries	1 cup	8.0
Pear (with skin)	1 medium	5.5
Apple (with skin)	1 medium	4.4
Banana	1 medium	3.0
Orange	1 medium	3.0

GRAINS	SERVING SIZE	TOTAL FIBER (GRAMS)
The grains group is high in B vitamins and several key minerals, including magnesium, which is involved in more than three hundred health-promoting actions in the body. Try to have 1 or 2 servings daily.		
Quinoa, cooked	1 cup	17.0
Bulgur wheat, cooked	1 cup	8.0
Barley, pearled, cooked	1 cup	6.0
Oatmeal, instant, cooked	1 cup	4.0
Brown rice, cooked	1 cup	3.0

SEEDS	SERVING SIZE	TOTAL FIBER (GRAMS)
Seeds pack a fiber punch in a tiny package. Have 1 or 2 servings daily.		
Chia seeds	1 ounce (2 tablespoons)	10.7
Flaxseeds	1 ounce (2 tablespoons)	8.5
Squash and pumpkin seeds	1 ounce (2 tablespoons)	5.0
Dried coconut (unsweetened)	1 ounce (2 tablespoons)	4.6
Chestnuts	1 ounce (2 tablespoons)	2.0

WATER IS LIFE FUEL

> Pure water is the
> world's first and
> foremost medicine.
>
> **—SLOVAKIAN PROVERB**

ABOUT FIFTEEN YEARS AGO, I signed up for a twelve-hour adventure race in Florida with a great friend of mine who is a beast of an athlete. The race was a combination of trail running, mountain biking, kayaking, and orienteering (finding your way to different checkpoints in the woods in total darkness—no GPS allowed, just good old-fashioned map and compass). When he mentioned the race, I was sold!

The fun started at seven p.m. If we didn't finish by seven the following morning, we'd be automatically disqualified. Everyone was required to cross all the checkpoints in a certain amount of time or risk being disqualified.

I can remember that night as if it were yesterday. I showed up with my backpack full of allowable gear—headlamp, waterproof matches, compass, and so forth. My friend and I were so pumped up that we couldn't wait for the race to begin.

The starting bell sounded, and we flew out of the starting line. About an hour into the race, my friend felt a cramp creeping into his left calf. Cramps can be dangerous because the sudden muscle pain can be so severe that an athlete could fall and risk serious injury. He drank some fluids (mostly water and electrolytes) and kept going.

An hour later, the cramp returned, but this time it was in his thigh. There was nothing he could do to make it go away. I could actually see the muscles of his thigh twisting under his skin into what seemed like excruciatingly painful knots. I was concerned about him, so

I asked about his hydration—few things can cripple an athlete more than dehydration. We slowed down for a little bit and he somehow managed to rehydrate (this is very rare and difficult once a race is under way). Some eight hours later, we finished the race at the top of our age group.

Water is critical whether you're an athlete or not, and dehydration can take you down. Water is life fuel. People can go for weeks without food, but the average person can't survive more than three days without water.

Water covers 71 percent of the earth's surface, makes up to 70 percent of your body, and is essential for the survival of every form of life. It is also the number one nutrient in our diets. Life just isn't possible without it.

THE MIRACLE NUTRIENT

Water does so many things in the body. For one, it kick-starts your metabolism. With the help of enzymes, it breaks down food into nutrients such as glucose, starches, fats, and protein for easy digestion. Water also helps the body metabolize stored fat. A German study found that drinking about a half gallon of cold water daily can help you burn up to an extra 50 calories a day. Researchers theorize that the metabolism surge comes from the extra effort needed to elevate the water's temperature to the temperature inside your body, 98.6°F. Drinking water can also help you feel full before a meal.

When your body has lots of water to work with, you feel energized. That's largely because adequate water acts as a solvent in which many of the body's nutrients, such as vitamins B and C, dissolve, making them available to the body. Water keeps your energy engine revved.

Many people who complain of fatigue are actually just dehydrated. Dehydration reduces blood flow to your organs, leaving you sluggish, and stresses your body. When your tissues don't obtain enough fluid, your cells start drawing water from your bloodstream, and your blood gets thicker. This places a strain on your heart, and you may feel weak or light-headed.

When you go plant-based, you'll be taking in a lot of fiber from food. (Remember Law #3?) Drinking enough water on a high-fiber diet is as important to your health as the fiber itself. That's because fiber absorbs a lot of water. As fiber winds its way through your digestive tract, expediting the removal of waste, it turns into a bulky mass. A lot of the fluid from this mass is withdrawn from your colon. If you are underhydrated, your stool may be dry and bowel movements may become difficult and painful. Water thus works as first aid for constipation.

Water is great for your joints. It makes up much of your synovial fluid, the "grease" in your joints, and cerebrospinal fluid, the shock-absorbing fluid between the vertebrae in your spine and around your brain. If your diet is water-deficient, even for a brief period, less of these essential fluids are available to protect your joint and spine health.

Your brain is composed of 70 to 80 percent fluids. You need those fluids for mental energy and overall brain power. In a

WATER CONTENT OF SELECTED PLANT FOODS

100%	Water
90 to 99%	Cantaloupe, strawberries, watermelon, lettuce, cabbage, celery, spinach, cucumbers, tomatoes, eggplant, squash, zucchini
80 to 89%	Apples, grapes, oranges, carrots, broccoli (cooked), pears, peaches, pineapple
70 to 79%	Bananas, avocados, potato (baked), kidney beans, corn (cooked)
60 to 69%	Other legumes
1 to 9%	Walnuts, peanuts (dry roasted), cereals

SOURCE: *USDA National Nutrient Database for Standard Reference, Release 21.*

study of subjects' abilities to perform mental exercises after dehydration induced by heat stress, a fluid loss of only 2 percent of body weight caused reductions of up to 20 percent in arithmetic ability, short-term memory, and the ability to visually track an object. Another study demonstrated that a minor loss of 1 percent of body mass as fluid led to impairments in both memory and attention. With that powerful proof, you should be motivated to stay well hydrated to keep your mental energy high and your focus sharp.

You might be surprised to learn that proper hydration may prevent cancer. One study found that people with urinary tract cancers (bladder, prostate, kidney, and testicle) drank significantly less fluid compared with healthy people. In another study, researchers discovered that women who drank more than five glasses of water a day had a 45 percent lower risk of colon cancer, compared with women who consumed two or fewer glasses a day. For men, the risk was cut by 32 percent when they drank more than four glasses a day versus one or fewer glasses a day.

Why does adequate water intake appear to help your body fight cancer? One theory holds that the more fluid you drink, the faster you flush toxins and carcinogenic substances out of your body, and the less chance there is for them to be reabsorbed into the body or concentrated long enough to cause tissue change.

No biological reaction or function in the body would be possible without water. It is required to cool the body, maintain muscle tone and skin tone, and provide a moist environment for ear, nose, and throat tissues. Water is needed to nourish cells, neurons, skin, and more. Water flushes out waste by dissolving excess salt and urea in the kidneys to pass out as urine, and to flush out toxins from your immune system, thus decreasing the risk of infections and viruses. Water helps your blood flow more fluidly to carry nutrients and oxygen through the body and also to prevent blood clots. It even makes you look more attractive by promoting a youthful glow and elasticity to your skin.

YOU CAN EAT YOUR WATER

Yes, you read that right. One of the advantages of plant-based eating—and one you don't hear much about—is that eating at least five servings a day of fruits and vegetables can provide about 20 percent of your daily water requirement. Basically, water-dense fruits and vegetables boost hydration naturally and leave you feeling fuller, in addition to supplying your body with luscious nutrients. The most succulent fruits are melons, watermelons, oranges, grapes, and apples. Other watery foods include carrots, cucumbers, radishes, and tomatoes.

HOW MUCH IS ENOUGH?

The quantity and quality of the fluids you drink daily are an important issue, both nutritionally and physiologically. Water will always be your best fluid choice. Unsweetened teas are great, too; so is water with lemon, cucumbers, or berries (if you like to "spike" your water with some extra flavor). Leave soda behind, skip the sugary teas, sugar-laden store-bought juices, lemonade, and alcohol. These all contain empty calories.

So how much water is enough? The Institute of Medicine suggests that men drink thirteen 8-ounce cups daily and women drink nine 8-ounce cups. Here are a few tips to help you manage your fluid intake throughout the day:

// Start your day with a glass of water with a little fresh lemon juice stirred in. This is good for alkalinity, digestion, and rehydration.

// Drink a glass of water with and between each meal to curb overeating and help you feel full between meals.

// Drink a glass of water before, during, and after exercise. Dehydration harms your exercise performance.

// Drink extra water when the weather is hot. Water the body loses through sweating must be replaced.

// Don't wait until you're thirsty to drink water; once you're thirsty, you are likely already dehydrated.

The best way to find out if you are getting enough water daily is to do a self-test.

First, you should be urinating regularly. For most people, it's normal to urinate six to eight times over a twenty-four-hour period. When your urine is practically colorless, that's a good sign that you're well hydrated. If you notice that the color of your urine is more like apple juice than lemonade, treat it as a warning bell to drink more water.

Besides the color of your urine, other signs of dehydration are dark circles or bags under your eyes, flaky skin or acne, a dry and red nose, headaches, and a dry mouth.

YOUR GREENPRINT
by Following Law #4

Besides the health benefits of adequate hydration, there is an environmental impact, depending on your water sources. Lots of energy is needed to produce the packaging for bottled and canned beverages. Plus, carbon is discharged into the environment during the manufacturing, transportation, and refrigeration of those bottles and cans. Most of them end up in landfills. Your "greenest" drink is good old filtered tap water. And rather than drink from plastic, use glass or stainless steel water bottles. You can increase your greenprint and lower your carbon footprint by making beverages such as coffee and tea at home instead of purchasing them in bottles or to-go cups.

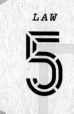

LAW

5

PROTECT YOUR HEART

> If you eat the
> standard Western
> diet that most
> people eat in
> the modern world,
> it's quite likely
> you will develop
> heart disease.
>
> —JOEL FUHRMAN

WHEN MY WIFE WAS PREGNANT with our first child, I remember the first time I heard his heartbeat ... *thump, thump, thump,* that precious first sign of life. It was a moment of profound emotion for me, and I fell in love.

Your own heart started to beat in your mother's womb. And it should continue to do so pretty much nonstop until you die. That's potentially billions of beats over a lifetime as your heart relaxes and fills with blood, then squeezes or contracts, pumping blood to and through all the parts of your body to nourish your entire system.

Your heart coexists with your life. You might be able to live with one kidney, or without your gallbladder, but your heart is inextricable from your life. When life ends, the heart fails; when the heart fails, life ends. When the heart ceases to function, it is most likely a result of abuse or lack of proper care. Our lifestyle, the food we eat, the attitudes we develop, and the activities we undertake—good or bad, these all affect the heart.

I don't mean to scare you, but any harm to your heart can be fatal. Heart disease kills about 610,000 people every year in the United States—that is about one in every four deaths. The greatest cause of death for women is heart disease, not cancer. Heart bypasses are performed on approximately 300,000 people each year. Every year, about 735,000 Americans have a heart attack. Of these people, 525,000 are first-time sufferers, but the remaining 210,000 have had a previous heart attack.

Risk to your heart can begin almost the moment you are born. Plaque starts accumulating inside the lining of your arteries (atherosclerosis) very early in life. In fact, plaque has been identified in the hearts of children as young as five years old, and a sizeable amount of buildup has been detected in the arteries of teenagers—the result of diets high in saturated fat and cholesterol. Thus, most American youths are at risk for heart disease.

Could any of this happen to you or your children?

If that question has invaded your thoughts, the answer depends on how you live your life. If you exercise regularly, eat mostly plant-based foods, and have an ideal body weight, you are less likely to suffer from heart problems.

The good news is, it's never too late to start making lifestyle changes to reduce your risk of heart disease. But which ones are best? Scores of books and articles pitch the "perfect" diet to prevent or reverse heart disease. The problem is that a lot of these plans just introduce confusion into the mix and offer no clear solution.

BUT THERE IS A CLEAR SOLUTION: plant-based eating. Before I jump into some powerful scientific proof, let me tell you about a friend of mine, Steve, a super-successful businessman who overcame enormous obstacles in life. His father wasn't often around, and when he was, he was a poor role model for Steve. He grew up in the wrong neighborhood, surrounded by drugs and alcohol, and his peer group was a bad influence. But armed with determination and an iron will, Steve decided he would be the master of his destiny, not a product of his environment.

Steve found success in his life, but as is often the case for successful people, he liked to indulge in various types of food and rarely had time to exercise. At age forty-five, he went to his physician for his routine annual physical, only to learn that he had dangerously high blood pressure and was on the verge of being diabetic.

We met for breakfast the day after his physical.

"How could this happen to me?" he asked, his head hung low. "I want to live a long life, and I've just started to have fun. But I don't want to depend on drugs or suffer their side effects. I'm willing to do whatever it takes."

PLANT PROTECTION FOR YOUR HEART

"It's simple," I said. "Go on a whole-food plant-based diet, and stick to it."

He had often heard me talking about plant-based eating, but until he had his health scare, he wasn't ready to really listen. Steve didn't mess around. He immediately went 100 percent plant-based and was more focused than I'd ever seen him.

Another friend asked him, "Man, are you really doing this plant-based thing?" His reply was as serious as it was comical: "You're damn right. I got a death sentence—high blood pressure and diabetes—but I said, 'No way, not me!'"

Four months later, Steve returned to his doctor for a follow-up visit, and his test results were nothing short of miraculous. His cholesterol was completely normalized, his blood pressure perfect, and his prediabetic condition was completely reversed.

How were these results possible, and why hadn't his doctor recommended this sort of diet right away? Well, I can't answer that, but I can say this: When it comes to two-word phrases, "plant-based" is a lot easier to hear than "bypass surgery" or, worse, "heart attack." It just so happens that plant-based living is the number one key to preventing—or even reversing—heart disease. This is fact—not me pushing my personal agenda, but rather me emphasizing the truth about how to control your manageable risk factors and take preventive dietary steps to lower your odds of a heart attack or stroke.

You may be reducing your consumption of beef burgers, but skipping Big Macs alone isn't enough to afford you substantial heart-healthy benefits from your diet. In a study published in the *Journal of the American College of Cardiology* in 2017, researchers examined more than two hundred thousand adults and reaffirmed the finding that adherence to a plant-based diet rich in whole grains, fruits, vegetables, nuts, and legumes was associated with a lower relative risk of coronary heart disease (CHD).

However, the study also noted that meatless diets that included substantial amounts of refined grains and sugar-sweetened beverages—basically junk food—were associated with higher risks of CHD. The key takeaway from this is to focus on the quality of the foods you're eating. For example, whole grains are much healthier for you than refined grains, because the refining process removes the dietary fiber, iron, and many B vitamins from the grains. Whole fruits are also better than fruit juices, because they contain healthy dietary fiber that has been stripped out in the juicing process.

If you have heart disease right now, you may be able to improve or alleviate your condition with a 100 percent plant-based diet. Researchers at the prestigious Cleveland Clinic tracked 198 patients and counseled them in plant-based nutrition. These patients had been diagnosed with cardiovascular disease (CVD) and were interested in transitioning to plant-based eating as a complement to their usual cardiovascular care. They were asked to eliminate dairy, fish, meat, and added oil from their diets.

Most of the volunteer patients with CVD responded well to counseling, and those who stayed on a plant-based diet for an average of 3.7 years had a low incidence of subsequent cardiac events. The researchers concluded that "plant-based nutrition has the potential for a large effect on the CVD epidemic." Or, as I like to say, a plant-based diet is your heart's best bodyguard!

HERE ARE SPECIFICS ON THE BEST CATEGORIES OF PLANT FOODS TO PROTECT YOUR HEART.

VEGETABLES // I love vegetables— their taste, how they change when you put them in the oven and roast them, and how they cohabitate so deliciously with grains, nuts, and seeds. Vegetables are magical— especially for your heart. Dark leafy greens, for example, are loaded with potassium, which helps control blood pressure, and antioxidants and phytochemicals to fight heart disease and other illnesses.

Leafy greens like kale, spinach, and collard greens contain nutrients that assist your body in creating new copies of the cells that line artery walls. Healthy, elastic arteries, in turn, produce ample nitric oxide, a beneficial molecule that keeps your blood vessels dilated and relaxed.

FRUIT // Does heart disease run in your family like it does in mine? Enjoy more fresh fruit. Research suggests that eating fruit (in addition to fresh veggies) may cut the risk of heart disease in people with genetic risks. Their power lies in the various heart-protective compounds they contain. One of these compounds is quercetin, a phytonutrient found in apples, grapes, cherries, and berries, as well as some vegetables, that has antioxidant and anti-inflammatory properties. And many fruits are potassium superstars, a mineral with the power to lower blood pressure. Vitamin C, an antioxidant vitamin common in fruits and some veggies, may protect against heart disease by relaxing arteries and stabilizing arterial plaque, thus preventing it from breaking off and causing a heart attack.

Then there's the avocado (yes, it's a fruit). Avocados are so powerfully heart-protective that even the FDA has agreed they can be labeled "heart-healthy." My reverence for avocados goes well beyond guacamole. I love this fruit so much that I even use it as the base for pies and puddings.

EXTRA-VIRGIN OLIVE OIL // Its beauty is that it comes packed with compounds that reduce inflammation of the arteries and decrease the formation of arterial plaque. Make this fat one of your main plant-based oils. A study from Greece, published in *Clinical Cardiology* in 2007, reported that the exclusive use of olive oil in cooking was linked to a 47 percent lower risk of acute coronary syndrome (sudden reduced blood flow to the heart), compared with not using olive oil.

WHAT ARE THE IDEAL

RECOMMENDATIONS
FOR CHOLESTEROL?

Medical authorities have established the following desirable ranges for cholesterol:

TOTAL
CHOLESTEROL
UNDER
200

LDL
CHOLESTEROL
UNDER
100

HDL
CHOLESTEROL
60
OR HIGHER

TRIGLYCERIDES
UNDER
150

VLDL
CHOLESTEROL
UNDER
30

GUIDELINES FOR CHOLESTEROL?

The 2015–2020 USDA Dietary Guidelines for Americans outline the following recommendations for keeping your body's cholesterol low:

CHOLESTEROL | Eat as little dietary cholesterol as possible (but there are no specific limits). Dietary cholesterol itself is only found in animal-based foods, including meat, dairy products, seafood, and egg yolks.

SATURATED FATS | Limit these fats, which are found mostly in meat and dairy foods, to less than 10 percent of the calories you consume per day.

UNSATURATED FATS | Replace saturated fats with unsaturated fats (mostly found in plant-based foods) as often as possible. There's no upper limit for healthy unsaturated fats.

TRANS FATS | Eat little to no synthetic trans fats, as they're associated with inflammation.

NUTS // Nuts have gotten a bad rap over the past few years, being touted as "high in fat" and calories. In reality, however, nuts eaten in moderation can have a variety of health benefits—including significantly improving your heart health.

A few recent studies reported by Harvard have indicated that if you regularly consume nuts, you could reduce your risk of heart attack and heart disease. These larger studies show consistent results—consuming nuts daily (or at least a few times per week) can reduce heart disease and heart attack risk by 30 to 50 percent. These recent studies have prompted the FDA to advise that a diet that includes 1 ounce of nuts per day can reduce the risk of heart disease.

So how, exactly, do nuts help you achieve better heart health? For one, they are a great source of unsaturated (good) fats, which can help reduce "bad" (LDL) cholesterol levels and raise "good" (HDL) cholesterol. Nuts are also a good source of omega-3 fatty acids, which can help calm erratic heart rhythms and reduce the risk of blood clots. Nuts are also a source of the essential amino acid arginine, which helps your body produce nitric oxide. In turn, nitric oxide relaxes your blood vessels to help lower your blood pressure. But that's not all—nuts are also a great source of vitamin E, folic acid, fiber, and potassium.

What about the calories in nuts? At an average 185 calories per ounce, adding nuts to your diet won't do much to help your health if they're not replacing a less healthy food—those calories can add up quickly. But by swapping in nuts for less healthy snacks, you'll be just fine.

Among the nuts that love your heart are pecans, pistachios, hazelnuts, almonds, and walnuts. So grab some nuts! Sprinkle them on cereal and salads, throw in a smoothie, or combine with dried fruit for a healthy snack. Your heart will thank you for it.

SEEDS // These are nutrition powerhouses. I love chia seeds and flaxseeds. Both give you omega-3 fats. Flaxseeds contain lignans, strong antioxidants, and cholesterol-lowering fiber.

One of my favorite seeds is quinoa. I've been cooking with it for more than fifteen years because I love its nutty flavor and light texture. Plus, it is packed full of protein and fiber, and contains all the essential amino acids our bodies need.

GRAINS // Various studies spotlight whole grains in heart disease prevention. In the 2000 Iowa Women's Health Study, women with the highest intakes of whole grains had 30 percent less risk of heart disease, compared with women who ate fewer whole grains. Many components of whole grains have heart-protecting benefits: Whole grains contain more heart-protective antioxidants than refined grains, and both oats and barley are super sources of beta-glucan, a fiber that lowers blood cholesterol and improves insulin sensitivity.

LEGUMES // Beans and legumes may give you more birthday candles. When researchers analyzed the diets of older adults in Japan, Greece, Sweden, and Australia, they found that the more legumes these folks ate, the longer they lived. And if you eat at least four servings of beans a week, you just might lower your risk of heart disease by 22 percent, according to a study of nearly ten thousand men and women in the United States. Beans are a treasure trove of many heart-protecting nutrients, including potassium, magnesium, folate, cholesterol-lowering fiber, and glucose-lowering resistant starches.

My parents are Cuban, so I was practically weaned on black beans, a staple in my culture. What's special about black beans is their high levels of antioxidants, particularly anthocyanin, a pigment that gives black and blue fruits, berries, and beans their color and health benefits. Black beans are rich in protein, fiber, zinc, copper, and molybdenum (a lesser-known but key mineral associated with longevity). Don't fear the gas that comes with eating beans. Start with small servings, and your body will adjust over time.

WHAT MEAT DOES TO YOUR HEART

Eating meat isn't so good for your heart. In 2012, scientists at the Harvard School of Public Health published data on more than 120,000 participants in their acclaimed Health Professionals Follow-Up Study and the Nurses' Health Study. After twenty-eight years, study participants who ate the most red meat (roughly two servings a day) had a 30 percent higher risk of dying than those who consumed the least (a serving a day or less).

This wasn't the first time a major study linked red meat to a shorter life span,

however. In 2009, the NIH-AARP Diet and Health Study reported results on half a million people. After ten years, those who ate the most red meat (about 5 ounces a day) were 30 percent more likely to die than those who consumed the least (about $2/3$ ounce a day). There are lots of other studies that point to the dangers of eating meat, so when you look at the whole picture, I'd say the evidence is very strong at this point. Eating too much meat may increase your risk of dying before your time. The medical recommendation limiting red meat intake is based on its saturated fat and cholesterol content, both of which increase artery-damaging LDL cholesterol levels in the blood. Red meat is one of the largest sources of saturated fat in the average American's diet. It's also important to avoid processed foods, other animal proteins, and dairy in order reduce your intake of saturated fat and cholesterol. Removing these foods from your diet protects the endothelial cells that line the walls of your arteries, and helps keep them from releasing compounds that constrict and clog your arteries.

THERE'S ANOTHER REASON TO CUT RED MEAT, EGGS, DAIRY, AND OTHER ANIMAL PROTEINS FROM YOUR DIET: These foods form more bad bacteria in your gut that churn out a compound called trimethylamine N-oxide (TMAO). TMAO creates inflammation that clogs your arteries.

I meet so many people who think it's hard to give up meat. It's not, and one of our Holy Name study participants, Ana, is proof. She's a medical and surgery oncology manager at a hospital in New Jersey.

SOON AFTER BEING SELECTED FOR THE STUDY, THE CHALLENGE WAS SET: Could she give up meat and animal foods and stick to a plant-based diet for the duration of the study? It would be a tough test for her, a Hispanic woman who has always devoured meat, chicken, eggs, and cheese and other dairy foods with carnivorous enthusiasm. And, like me, she's a self-proclaimed foodie!

"I thought it would be difficult and I'd be hungry, and how would I get my protein? But I stayed with it." Like many people I've worked with, Ana was overfocused on protein at first—when she needed to be concerned about fiber. Her digestive system was sluggish and bathroom trips were every other day—and she knew that these issues had to be resolved.

After she went entirely plant-based during the study, they were. And no wonder—Ana was eating a lot more fiber, thanks to beans, fresh vegetables, quinoa, brown rice, and fruits. During her vegan journey, Ana discovered that it was easy to adapt her native cuisine to plant-based dishes: from quinoa and brown rice for white rice to various tomato-based vegan dishes. Bonus: Plants have plenty of protein. Slowly but surely, her husband began to try—and like—many of her plant-based dishes.

Ana noticed something very common when you go plant-based: the diet peeled inches off her body. "All my clothes, including jeans, got looser and looser."

One of the nicest surprises was better blood-sugar control. This was important to Ana since people of Hispanic and Latino origin are at high risk for developing type 2 diabetes, a condition characterized by high blood glucose levels caused by either a lack of insulin or the body's inability to use insulin efficiently. Type 2 diabetes develops most often in middle-aged and older adults but can appear in young people, says the American Diabetes Association.

Ana's hemoglobin A1C—a measurement of diabetes risk—moved into the normal range. Heart health measures, such as LDL cholesterol and blood pressure, also normalized. So did her liver function enzymes.

The most important lesson Ana learned was that "if I eat meat, it really messes me up. I can feel how I am hurting my body if I veer off the diet."

So you might want to think twice before you toss that burger or steak on the grill.

YOUR GREENPRINT
by Following Law #5

Eating more fruits and vegetables (four or five servings daily) decreases your risk of heart disease by 17 percent, according to a 2013 *American Journal of Clinical Nutrition* study.

LAW

6

TAKE CARE OF YOUR MIND

> One of the hardest
> things you will
> ever have to do is
> to grieve the loss
> of a person who is
> still alive.
>
> **—UNKNOWN**

WE'VE ALL HAD THE EXPERIENCE of walking around in a parking lot only to forget where we parked our car, right? Hey, it happens. But it sure makes you think about your powers of recall. Is this a normal bout of forgetfulness or something more sinister? Is dementia setting in? Should you be concerned about your brain fitness?

For those of you who would like to improve your memory and prevent one of the scariest diseases around—Alzheimer's—there's strong proof that plant-based eating keeps your cognitive powers as sharp as possible, and the sooner you start eating plant-based, the better.

A little background: Alzheimer's disease, which involves the breakdown of neuronal communication, is currently the sixth leading cause of death in the United States. Ten percent of people age sixty-five and older have Alzheimer's, and the incidence in this age range in America is expected to increase from 48 million to 88 million by the year 2050.

The standard treatment for Alzheimer's disease consists of a few medications, which only help to slow the progression of the disease, not cure it. Therefore, it is critical to find more effective methods to prevent the development of this dreaded disease. I have been keenly

LONGEVITY

& PLANT-BASED EATING

HAVE YOU EVER READ ABOUT "BLUE ZONES"?

A Blue Zone is a region of the world where people commonly enjoy active lives—mentally and physically—past the age of one hundred years. Scientists and health professionals have classified these longevity "hot spots" around the world by life practices that result in higher than normal longevity. In fact, Loma Linda is currently the only Blue Zone in the entire United States.

A good read on this topic is Dan Buettner's book *The Blue Zones*, which outlines the healthy habits, diets, and cultural and familial values each longevity society upholds. Through interviews, it also provides glimpses into how and why these people live to be one hundred years old or older. The main Blue Zones are the island of Sardinia, Italy; the Nicoya Peninsula, Costa Rica; Loma Linda, California; and Okinawa, Japan.

Although the dietary patterns of Blue Zones vary, the common denominator is that folks in these areas eat a high percentage of plant-based whole foods that are naturally low in fat. For example, in Okinawa, Japan—the Blue Zone thought to have greatest longevity and freedom from chronic diseases—roughly 9 percent of an Okinawan's calories come from protein and 85 percent come from carbohydrates. In fact, grains and legumes were by far the biggest staples of the Okinawan diet, followed by sweet potatoes.

And how did all these foods affect health? Rates of heart disease are 80 percent lower compared with those in the United States. Rates of breast and prostate cancer were 75 percent lower, and dementia 67 percent lower.

What's the takeaway here? Any diet that doesn't repeatedly emphasize this one simple step—*eat more plants and fewer animal foods*—is missing the mark in terms of life span.

As they say, an apple a day . . .

interested in the role of diet—in particular, the influence of a plant-based diet—in the prevention of Alzheimer's. Nature has gifted us with a plethora of plants—fruits, vegetables, and nuts that make our planet beautiful and also give us the best nutrition we can possibly get. They contain a diverse array of neuroprotective nutrients that may play a pivotal role in the prevention and, one day, perhaps even the cure of various neurodegenerative diseases such as Alzheimer's.

In my review of the science, I found that the consumption of leafy green vegetables, fruits such as blueberries, and spices such as saffron or turmeric have brain-protective properties. On the other hand, eating lots of saturated fats and sugars is linked to the development of Alzheimer's. Let me briefly run through some eye-opening science with you. When examining the link between diet and cognitive function, one study found that people whose midlife diets were characterized as healthy (high in plant-based foods, low in saturated fats, and so forth) had a lower risk of dementia and Alzheimer's disease later in life compared with people with unhealthy diets rich in meat and dairy foods. The difference was staggering: People who ate the healthiest had an 86 to 90 percent decreased risk of dementia and a 90 to 92 percent decreased risk of Alzheimer's disease compared with people whose diets were largely meat-based.

Another study followed participants for twenty to thirty years and revealed that people with higher cholesterol levels in midlife had a significantly higher risk

(1.5 times higher) of developing Alzheimer's disease and dementia later in life.

Writing in the *Journal of the American College of Nutrition* in 2016, researchers found that "the most important dietary link to Alzheimer's disease appears to be meat consumption, with eggs and high-fat dairy also contributing."

Why is that? It has to do largely with animal-based saturated fat, found in butter, cheese, and meat.

Here's what's going on, according to a study published online in the June 17, 2013, edition of *JAMA Neurology*: Saturated fat not only clogs blood vessels in the brain and triggers damaging inflammation, but also deprives the brain of a protein it needs to protect itself from the accumulation of toxic beta-amyloid plaque, which is a hallmark of Alzheimer's disease. In other research news, Brigham and Women's Hospital in Boston published the results of a study that found that among more than six thousand older women, those who ate the greatest amount of saturated fat over a period of just four years were 60 percent more likely to have significant mental decline than those who ate the least amount.

What we put into our mouth makes a big difference to our brain health (and the health of our other organs). To protect your brain and slash your risk of dementia, eat plenty of whole grains, legumes, and fresh fruits and vegetables. These foods are packed with healthy chemicals called polyphenols.

Polyphenols are a type of antioxidant (and we all know how beneficial antioxidants are to our health) that fight chronic inflammation. Inflammation is the underlying cause of many age-related diseases, including Alzheimer's. Polyphenols tend to concentrate in the brain, and consuming polyphenols is associated with lower rates of age-related cognitive decline.

After my first year of eating plant-based, I had one of the most meaningful events on my plant-based journey. I went in for my physical and routine blood tests, and when the results came back, my inflammation markers were so low, they were barely detectable. My doctor asked what I was doing differently, and I was happy to tell him that my shift to a plant-based diet had been more effective than I had ever dreamed possible.

If you want to boost your brain health, have laser-sharp focus all day long, and prevent age-related mental decline and Alzheimer's, follow this law now!

I SUGGEST THAT YOU:

// Get off saturated fats and trans fats. That means stop eating meat, dairy, and cheese—and all processed foods.

// Replace meats and dairy products with vegetables, beans and legumes, fruits, and whole grains.

// Get vitamin E from foods like seeds, nuts, leafy green veggies, and whole grains, rather than from supplements. It helps protect damage to your arteries, including those that go into the brain.

// Add a special boost to protect your brain and nervous system in the form of berries (blueberries, raspberries, strawberries). Berries have been shown

to have a protective effect due to their high flavonoid content. Flavonoids are another group of natural compounds found only in plants, and research indicates they might be neuroprotective.

// Eat colorful plant-based foods at every meal, since these foods are brain-protective.

// Exercise regularly, too, since working out keeps your brain young and your thinking sharp.

All these actions are choices—just as eating animal-based foods and processed foods are choices. Ultimately, these choices become habits. Over the past fifteen years, I have cultivated the habit of eating the gorgeous, bountiful, beautiful, vibrant foods that the earth gives us. I eat fruits and vegetables that maximize my physical and mental health. I eat foods that cut my risk not only of Alzheimer's but also of diabetes and heart disease. These are my habits, and they are building my health and my success in every part of my life.

Why not start cultivating the good habits now?

It is still not too late to reverse the effects of choices you made when you either didn't know better or didn't care as much. If this describes you, and you want to take care of your mind, switching to plant-based eating is the place to start. With these easy dietary tweaks, you'll be helping your health, not harming it. I did it. And you can, too.

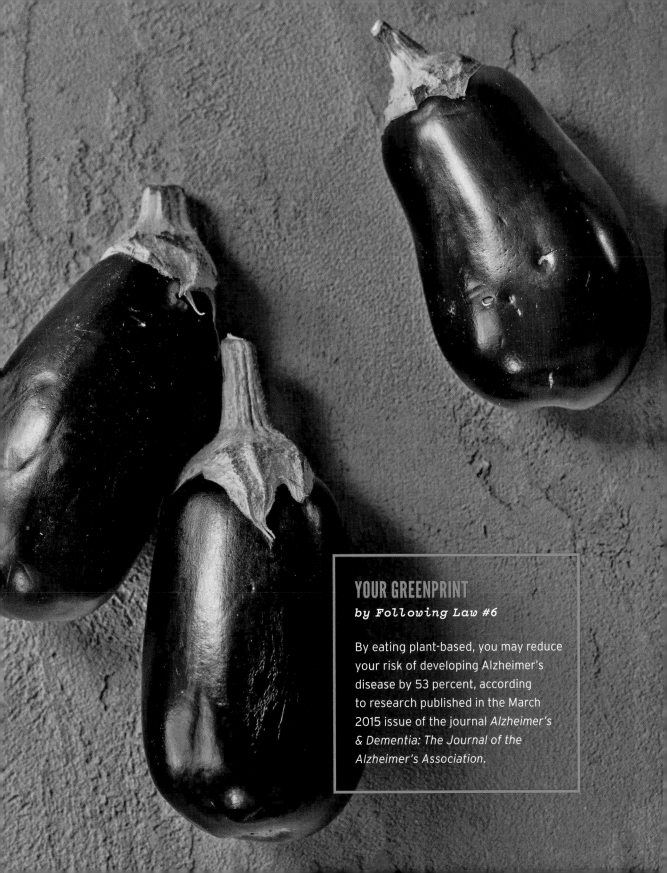

YOUR GREENPRINT
by Following Law #6

By eating plant-based, you may reduce your risk of developing Alzheimer's disease by 53 percent, according to research published in the March 2015 issue of the journal *Alzheimer's & Dementia: The Journal of the Alzheimer's Association.*

FAST FOR HEALTH AND LONGEVITY

The best
of all
medicines
are resting
and fasting.

—BENJAMIN FRANKLIN

I JOINED THE "INTERMITTENT FASTING" movement several years ago during a search for additional solutions for clients who needed to lose 50 pounds or more. That's about the time when science was reporting the benefits of intermittent fasting for weight loss, disease prevention, and longevity.

This law may sound like a new law to you, but fasting has been incorporated into various religions and cultures practically since the dawn of time. Historically, people fasted to increase their spiritual progress and deepen their faith. Now that you see how this law works, you have the opportunity to make it a habit—and earn the rewards of a healthier, longer life.

Intermittent fasting is something we practice already, even if we don't know it. It's called sleeping—going with as many as sixteen hours without food between dinner and breakfast. That's the easiest form of fasting to do, and the body burns fat for energy during that time period. With intermittent fasting, between 85 and 100 percent of weight lost is pure fat.

Basically, intermittent fasting is defined as an eating pattern in which you alternate periods of eating and fasting. The focus is on the timing of consumption of your healthy meals. There are variations on the intermittent fasting theme. One is the 24-hour fast (going without food entirely for one day); another is eating regularly for five days, followed by two days of fasting. Then there's fasting once a week. There's the alternate-day modified fast, too, in which every other day, you eat only one meal with maybe 30 percent of your normal (non-fasting) daily calories.

Because intermittent fasting has become so popular and useful for weight control, I was eager to read the results of a study by Valter Longo, funded by the National Institute on Aging and the National Cancer Institute. He incorporated plant-based nutrition—which piqued my interest considerably—in his research. This study shed further light on the fact that intermittent fasting—actually, just eating very lightly—can help people lose weight. Those who ate a special low-calorie, plant-based diet five days a month not only lost weight, but lowered their cholesterol, blood pressure, and body fat measurements. The rest of the month, they could eat whatever they wanted. This particular diet provided 750 to 1,100 calories a day from plant-based food bars, soup packets, and teas.

On average, dieters dropped around 5 pounds after three months on the diet. They also showed less evidence of inflammation, which is linked with cancer, heart disease, and obesity. They got better control of their blood sugar, too, which is a risk factor for diabetes.

Intrigued, I began reading other studies on intermittent fasting and discovered how it might make us live longer. Harvard researchers, for example, showed how this form of fasting can increase life span, slow aging, and improve health by altering the activity of mitochondria, the little energy factories inside our cells that are fundamental to cell aging. Mitochondria exist in networks that dynamically change shape according to energy demand. Their capacity to do so declines with age.

Using nematode worms, an organism useful for studying longevity because it only lives for two weeks, the study found that intermittent fasting manipulates those mitochondrial networks to keep them in a "youthful" state. In addition, researchers found that these youthful networks increase life span by communicating with organelles called peroxisomes to modulate fat metabolism.

Also, intermittent fasting helps autophagy. If you haven't heard of autophagy, it's time you did. It is a new word circulating in science and wellness circles, and with good reason. Autophagy, which translates to "eating of self," is a self-cleaning mechanism of our cells. Think of it as a housekeeper who sweeps away cellular debris, breaks it apart, and recycles the parts into fuel. Without this self-cleansing, cells would be overcome with damaged, unnecessary fragments and pathogens, and eventually malfunction and

INTERMITTENT FASTING

1

It helps to **KEEP YOUR BLOOD SUGAR STABLE** in the body, reducing insulin resistance in the process, which is great for preventing prediabetes.

2

It gives your digestion a much-needed rest and triggers important cellular repair processes, such as removing waste from cells. This helps to **REDUCE INFLAMMATION**, too.

3

It helps you **CONSUME FEWER CALORIES**. Instead of running on fuel from the food you just ate, fasting lets your body tap into fat storage for energy. Thus, it's a great way to lose weight and belly fat.

4

While long-term fasting can actually cause a drop in your metabolism, intermittent fasting **ACCELERATES METABOLISM.**

5

It **STIMULATES YOUR BRAIN** by promoting the growth of brain cells. Also, it helps decrease the risk of developing neurodegenerative diseases like Parkinson's and Alzheimer's.

6

It **STRENGTHENS YOUR IMMUNE SYSTEM** by boosting the body's production of new white blood cells, which equip the body to fight various infections and fend off invaders.

7

It produces an **ANTIAGING** benefit on the body.

die. Why should you care about autophagy? Well, here's why:

// It regulates metabolism and fat loss.

// It affects energy levels.

// It helps build and restore muscle.

// When autophagy isn't working properly, cells can't efficiently fight off certain diseases, including cancer, diabetes, muscular dystrophy, Alzheimer's, and Parkinson's.

// It may influence inflammation and your immune system.

// It slows the aging process.

// It aids brain function and reduces neurological cellular breakdown.

Eating slows down autophagy, so it stands to reason that intermittent fasting—those short periods of time when you don't eat—would support this process. Put another way, intermittent fasting ramps autophagy into action. In fact, autophagy may explain much of the positive research behind intermittent fasting.

Based on this knowledge, my experience, and these studies combined, I became a strong advocate of intermittent fasting, since it helps you live longer—and in a slimmer, fitter body!

HOW INTERMITTENT FASTING WORKS

Where food is concerned, your body goes into one of two states—the "fed" state and the "fast" state. When you start the process of eating and digesting, your body enters the fed state. After you've finished eating, your body stays in the fed state for 3 to 5 hours, and generally you don't feel hungry (especially if your meals are plant-based). In the fed state, your body's insulin level goes up to get glucose into your cells for fuel. When your insulin levels are elevated, there's no need for your body to burn fat for energy.

However, after 3 to 5 hours, the fed state is over, and your insulin levels begin to drop. After dinner, when you go for 10 to 16 hours without food, your body starts to burn the energy stored in your fat. As long as you're eating, your body is using up the energy from that food but not burning stored fat. But when you fast, your body first burns up any surplus sugar, then taps into stored fat for energy. The longer you can stretch the gap between dinner and breakfast, the better your body can burn fat. For example, if you have your dinner at six p.m., try to have breakfast later the next day, like at ten a.m. By following this timetable, you have a 16-hour gap of potential fat-burning between meals.

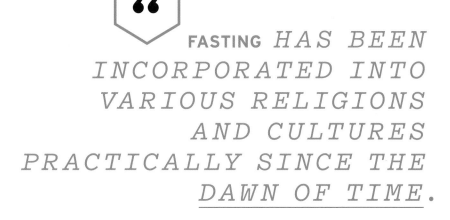

> *FASTING* *HAS BEEN INCORPORATED INTO VARIOUS RELIGIONS AND CULTURES PRACTICALLY SINCE THE DAWN OF TIME.*

TRY IT!

I advise my clients who want to try intermittent fasting to fast in the evenings several times a week. They don't eat for 16 hours after dinner, then break their fast with a late breakfast the next day, and consume their other meals within a 8-hour window after breakfast.

Intermittent fasting will work well for you if you're used to skipping meals or if you feel like you're too busy to eat. Don't be afraid to try it—skip a meal here and there if you're up to the challenge and want to take advantage of the benefits intermittent fasting offers.

When you do eat, choose quality foods such as fruits, vegetables, and whole grains that have lots of nutrients relative to their calories. They will fill you up, so you won't feel deprived or hungry during your fasting period.

YOUR GREENPRINT
by Following Law #7

You'll help your body stay naturally thin and fit. A systematic review of forty studies found that intermittent fasting was effective for weight loss, with a typical loss of 7 to 11 pounds over ten weeks, according to a 2015 report published in *Molecular and Cellular Endocrinology*.

LAW

THINK ABOUT THE EARTH BEFORE YOU EAT

> The environment is where we all meet; where all have a mutual interest; it is the one thing all of us share.
>
> **—LADY BIRD JOHNSON**

FOR A VERY LONG TIME, Americans believed we had the world's healthiest and safest diet. We worried little about this diet's effect on the planet. Nor did we worry about its ability to endure—that is, its sustainability.

But now we've come to recognize our Western diet is unhealthy and unsafe. Modern agriculture is ruining our soil and poisoning natural habitats, and animals are produced for food as if they were widgets. It would be hard to devise a more wasteful, damaging, unsustainable system.

Now we're smarter. We know we can make food choices every day that have a significant impact not only on our bodies but also on our planet—and we don't have to overhaul our lives to do it. We can create important and sustainable food habits that will make a huge difference on our personal greenprint—and our health. Here's how to do something positive for the planet by thinking about the earth before we eat.

BECOME A "LOCAVORE"

The food you eat comes from somewhere. Have you really thought about its origins? I'm betting that every week, you shop at the same store or two, hit the same aisles, and come home with the same products. And most of the food you're buying has been processed hundreds or thousands of miles away and preserved with chemicals so it can sit on trucks and storage shelves for months until you take it home. Naturally this makes a lot of food unhealthy, but you can combat this by becoming a locavore.

Merriam-Webster's defines a "locavore" as "one who eats foods grown locally whenever possible." Joining this class of food consumers is really important—for your health and for the planet.

For one thing, eating locally reduces the number of miles that food travels, which reduces greenhouse gas emissions. Eating locally produced foods also helps preserve local jobs, because farmers can sell their products within their communities.

Locally grown food is healthier. Crops are harvested at their peak, making them better for you. The shorter the time it takes produce to get from the field to your table, the less likely it is that nutrients will be lost. The Institute of Food Research reports that fresh vegetables transported long distances lose up to 45 percent of their nutritional value between the time they are harvested and the time they're stocked in a grocery store.

Another huge benefit of local produce is that it tastes better. After I tasted local tomatoes, for example, other tomatoes just didn't have the same flavor. When you love how a veggie tastes, you're going to eat more of it.

Local food preserves the land and wildlife. When farmers get paid more for their products by marketing locally, they're less likely to sell farmland for development. Well-managed farms conserve soil fertility, protect water resources, and keep carbon from the atmosphere. These farms provide a patchwork of fields, woods, and ponds that provide habitats for wildlife.

SHOP AT FARMERS' MARKETS

My favorite shopping location is my local farmers' market. You can find farmers' markets all over the place, and they are a wonderful way to explore the seasonal and local offerings where you live. Making a trip to the farmers' market part of your weekly routine is fun for you and fun for your family. If you see something unfamiliar at the farmers' market, just ask what it is! Whoever is running the stand will probably have good ideas about how you can prepare it at home.

Food sold at farmers' markets tends to be seasonal. Seasonal foods are not cultivated in artificial conditions, such as heated greenhouses. Nor are they grown hundreds of miles away, harvested prematurely, and shipped long distances. They are more sustainable for the planet, because fewer resources and less energy are required to grow and ship them.

By purchasing directly from a local farmer, you're strengthening the time-honored ties between eater and grower. Knowing farmers provides insight into the seasons, the land, and your food. Involve your kids, too, and you give them the opportunity to learn about nature, nutrition, and agriculture.

CONSIDER CSAs

Although some of us could take a trip to the farmers' market on a regular basis, for others, it's just not feasible. A great alternative is to participate in a CSA (community-supported agriculture) program. It is a wonderful way to get involved with local farming and connect with local growers to get fresh, local goods, all while supporting your community's economy and one of our most important industries—agriculture. CSAs are big in the summertime, because that's when harvests come in.

Basically, a CSA is a contract between you and a local grower in which you provide them with income in exchange for a portion of their crop. You pay the grower a fee, and the grower commits to a weekly delivery of produce (or you can arrange to pick it up). Depending on how much you spend, you may receive a small, medium, or large box of fresh produce each week. You may be able to customize your box to include or exclude certain fruits or veggies. It's the best of both worlds—you get fresh veggies, and the grower gets a regular source of income.

CSAs are a little like a stock investment. A farmer issues a certain number of "shares" to consumers. Those shares generally consist of a box of vegetables. You purchase a share, and in return receive a box of seasonal produce each week throughout the farming season. CSAs thus differ from vegetable delivery services. Vegetable delivery simply means that you buy vegetables like you would in a grocery store, and the supplier (usually a grocer) delivers them to your doorstep.

If possible, try to find an organic CSA, so that you have access to produce free of pesticides and other harmful chemicals. And find one with an appealing selection of items.

To get started, find out if there are CSAs in your area by looking online or checking the Resources on page 297.

GO ORGANIC

Organic isn't just some trendy fad. The way food is grown impacts our environment and our health. That's because organic food is not grown with chemical pesticides and fertilizers. Eating organic ensures (as defined by law) that your foods are produced without growth hormones and GMOs, too.

It's not hard to imagine why choosing organic produce would be good for you, but many people still don't choose to eat organic. However, when you really consider the statistics, you'll find that the reasons to go organic keep adding up while the excuses not to fall by the wayside. So why is organic so much better than the alternative?

BENEFIT #1:
MORE NUTRIENTS

A host of scientific studies have shown that organic produce offers higher concentrations of nutrients and lower concentrations of pesticides. Specifically, food grown without traditional pesticides will be richer in antioxidants and lower in cadmium (a heavy metal commonly left after pesticide application).

If you're thinking, *Well, it's probably not a significant difference,* then this statistic will stick out: Organic blueberries are 50 percent higher in anthocyanins (the compound that gives them color and contains antioxidants) than their conventionally grown counterparts.

BENEFIT #2:
NO GMOs

In order for a product to be labeled "USDA Organic," it cannot be grown from genetically modified organisms (GMOs). No studies have shown a health benefit to consuming genetically modified foods, and a few studies have indicated that there might be long-term health risks. Like trans fats, we might not know what the true health risks of consuming genetically modified foods are for many years, and by then the damage will have been done.

BENEFIT #3:
NO PESTICIDES

There are more than four hundred different kinds of pesticides alone used in traditional (nonorganic) farming, which requires more energy, more water, and depletes soil fertility. As a result, our bodies are being robbed of the very nutrients we seek for total wellness and needlessly exposed to the dangerous effects of these methods. Avoiding foods high in pesticides can also help reduce the risks of certain disease, too, including Alzheimer's, Parkinson's, and endometriosis.

Although acceptable pesticide levels are set by the USDA, and fruits and veggies are typically washed prior to their arrival at your local supermarket, many can still hold residual levels of harmful chemicals. In fact, up to 65 percent of produce can still contain pesticides. But which types are the worst offenders?

Every year, the Environmental Working Group (EWG) identifies the twelve foods with the highest levels of pesticides. These are called the "Dirty Dozen." Here is the EWG's latest Dirty Dozen:

1 // Strawberries

2 // Spinach

3 // Nectarines

4 // Apples

5 // Grapes

6 // Peaches

7 // Cherries

8 // Pears

9 // Tomatoes

10 // Celery

11 // Potatoes

12 // Sweet bell peppers

Near the top of the list, apples are by far the worst offenders—with a whopping 99 percent of conventional apples testing positive for some type of pesticide residue. Grapes, a fan favorite with kids, can have up to fifteen types of pesticides on the single grape, something all parents should be aware of.

On the far side of the spectrum, many thick-skinned types of produce, including pineapple, mangoes, and eggplant, have lower levels of pesticides. Choosing produce lower on the list can be an alternative if pesticide-free plant foods are not readily available or affordable. If you have to purchase produce from the list, make sure you wash it thoroughly before eating it. Removing the peel can also help reduce pesticide residue.

Going organic is ultimately the best way to reduce your exposure to dangerous chemicals. But if you can't find organic options in the produce section, head over to the frozen foods aisle and look for organic frozen strawberries, peaches, and other foods.

Chemical pesticides are harmful to their surroundings, can get into groundwater, permanently damage the soil they leech into, and can have long-term effects on the body. Organic foods that reduce the use of pesticides and use natural deterrents (like good bugs) are a better alternative.

BENEFIT #4:
BETTER FOR THE ENVIRONMENT

If there's one reason to choose a meat-free, organic lifestyle, it's to save the planet! A colossal amount of chemicals is used to treat nonorganic produce, and the long-term damage to the surrounding soil should be a major cause for concern. Besides preventing the leeching of synthetic pesticides into

GMOs

There's a heated debate going on about genetically modified organisms (GMOs). Are they healthy? Should we be eating GMO foods? What are they doing to the environment?

FOR PERSPECTIVE, IT IS IMPORTANT TO UNDERSTAND WHAT, PRECISELY, A GMO IS

Genetic modification occurs when genes from one organism are injected into a fruit or vegetable in a lab. The result is a genetically modified organism. This process creates combinations of plant, animal, bacteria, and virus genes that do not occur in nature or through traditional crossbreeding methods.

Genetic modifications are often performed to make a fruit or vegetable more hardy and drought resistant, or impervious to the application of specific pesticides and herbicides, namely glyphosate, made by Monsanto and found in its Roundup products.

Glyphosate, by the way, is not "just" an herbicide. It was first patented as a mineral chelator. Chelators *restrain nutrients,* which makes them physiologically unavailable for your body. So there may be a key mineral in a plant food, but if it's chelated with glyphosate,

your body can't absorb it—you might as well be eating a little chunk of gravel. Of course, health problems are bound to arise if you're consistently eating foods from which your body cannot extract critical nutrients and minerals.

Glyphosate is *also* patented as an *antibiotic* that fights bacteria. Unfortunately, like all antibiotics, it kills off vitally important beneficial soil bacteria and human gut bacteria required for good health along with the bad bacteria it was intended to knock out.

GMOs that are heavily sprayed with glyphosate have lower nutrient quality than organic foods. They also contain high amounts of pesticides with documented harmful health effects, along with unfamiliar, and therefore highly allergenic, proteins.

Large population studies reveal that the increased usage of glyphosate correlates with an identical rise in over thirty human diseases.

I realize all these facts are startling, but there is a very easy way to avoid GMO foods: Eat organic produce, which by definition is not genetically modified, or look for "GMO-free" on food labels.

GENETICALLY MODIFIED CROPS COME WITH SOME POTENTIALLY PROBLEMATIC ENVIRONMENTAL CHALLENGES

CROP CONTAMINATION

Pollen from GM crops and trees can contaminate nearby crops, trees, and wild plants through cross-pollination (the exception is soy, which does not cross-pollinate).

TOXICITY

Studies have shown that pesticide-producing crops contaminate nearby streams, possibly affecting aquatic life. Toxic residues are left in the soil by GM crops, and nutrients are not returned to the soil.

HARM TO BENEFICIAL INSECTS

Beneficial insects include bees and butterflies. Bees are important pollinators of many food crops but are unfortunately extremely endangered by modern agricultural techniques, such as GM crops. Bees can transport pesticides, herbicides, and DNA through the air into the environment. Monarch butterflies are specifically at risk from GM maize. In addition to bees and butterflies, birds are also at risk.

SUPER WEEDS

As weeds adapt to herbicides, they develop resistance and evolve into "super weeds." When this happens, farmers have to use even more toxic poisons, such as 2,4-D (a major ingredient in Agent Orange), than they use on crops. GMO-contaminated super weeds can also become invasive in natural ecosystems.

WATER POLLUTION

The irrigation systems used to water GM foods carry all these problems into our water sources, exposing insects and animals to toxicity.

Always stay informed on the food you are eating, and the way modern agricultural techniques are affecting our plants and our planet. This is yet another effective way of applying this law.

the soil and water, organic farming helps to promote the health of surrounding wildlife who don't find that their food and water sources are contaminated.

Additionally, organic farming methods ensure that the soil retains its nutrients, so there's no need for fertilizers. Farmers also use natural methods of planting (such as mixed crops) to help the soil feed the plants.

Finally, since organic produce does not use chemicals to maintain freshness, a lot of organic food is sold locally—so there is a significant reduction in carbon emissions to get your food to market. Even better, find a farm close to home and pick up your own fruits and vegetables!

BENEFIT #5:
TASTES GREAT!

Many types of store-bought produce are treated with a "sealer," which retains freshness as the produce moves from the field, through processing, onto a truck or plane, and finally to your local market's shelves. These sealers often affect the taste of your produce. Additionally, the higher antioxidant levels in organic fruits and veggies make them taste better.

Plant foods are great—but even greater when they are organically grown, for our sake and the planet's.

GROW YOUR OWN

The organic food movement has made having a backyard garden popular again. When you grow your own fruits and vegetables, you have total control. Other than sunlight and water, no chemicals are needed, and your food is 100 percent organic.

If you don't see yourself out in the backyard with a hoe and trowel, or you live in an apartment or condo, you can try growing a container garden. Many vegetables happily grow in containers. Herbs, for example, particularly basil, rosemary, mint, and thyme, are easy container plants, and most only require a sunny spot by your window and regular watering.

Sprouts are super easy to grow. Try sprouting the seeds of broccoli, radishes, mung beans, lentils, and alfalfa. Simply place the seeds in a mesh-covered jar, fill with filtered water, and set aside to soak. Drain the soaking water and rinse the seeds twice a day—morning and evening—without removing them from the jar to promote germination. Keep the seeds between 50°F and 70°F until they sprout. After sprouting, use them right away—on salads, sandwiches, or wraps.

Try vertical gardening, too, in which you grow veggies in a container but train them to grow upward on a wall or trellis, or in a special planter. Veggies suitable for vertical gardening include vining squash, tomatoes, beans, cucumbers, pumpkin, and peas.

Growing vegetables at home from seed also saves money. And gardening can be a great family activity.

Planting a seed, nurturing its growth, and experiencing its beautiful expression in full bloom promotes a healthy relationship with all living things. In gardening, you can maintain a conscious connection to the earth.

too much, freeze it or incorporate it into soups and casseroles. Choose whole foods over processed, because packaged stuff not only takes more energy to produce but contributes to packaging waste as well. Not only that, but most packaged foods are only going to derail your weight loss goals.

By embracing Law #8, you renew your relationship with the earth and nurture yourself with wholesomeness by eating the plant-based foods that Nature offers. And that nurturing relationship is one of the most important connections on earth.

WASTE NOT

Did you know there is more food in our landfills than any other single material? It's true. In 2012, the Environmental Protection Agency reported that there was more than 36 million tons of food waste. Rotting food gives off a lot of methane, one of the greenhouse gases associated with global warming.

Adopt a no-waste mind-set by planning weekly menus and buying only as much produce as you know your family will eat (our meal planner is a wonderful resource for this: mealplanner.22daysnutrition.com). In other words, no bulk buying! If you do buy or cook

YOUR GREENPRINT
by Following Law #8

You will leave the smallest carbon footprint. Researchers at Loma Linda University have reported that plant eaters generate a 41.7 percent smaller volume of greenhouse gases than meat eaters do.

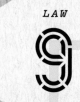

LOVE FOOD THAT LOVES YOU BACK

> Don't eat anything
> your great-great
> grandmother
> wouldn't recognize
> as food.
>
> —MICHAEL POLLAN

I LOVE FOOD: the smell, the taste, different food combinations, the experience of sitting down to a delicious dinner with my family and close friends. I'm an incurable experimenter with food and all the subtle and not-so-subtle variations accomplished with herbs and spices. These things are truly my passion, and they're glorious.

Food can certainly be seductive. We turn to food because it comforts us. While we're lusting after food, we're not thinking about how our clothes will stop fitting, our faces are going to break out, and our stomachs are going to bloat, or how we might get heart disease or diabetes.

Such conditions have serious consequences in terms of our lives. There are global consequences, too: There are more overweight people than hungry people on the planet, by a margin of at least several hundred million. And things are getting worse. The Centers for Disease Control and Prevention projects that by the middle of the twenty-first century, a stunning and devastating one in three people globally will have diabetes. If you eat whatever you want, whenever you want, as much as you want, neither your weight nor your health will be what you wish them to be.

When I was a little kid, I had an epiphany about food. One morning on my way to school, I ate a pastry. I didn't think much about it—until I got an angry rash on my arm right afterward. I tried to ignore it, but it kept getting worse. It itched, and my arm swelled up. I couldn't focus on my schoolwork. I went to the school nurse. She asked me if I had any allergies, and I knew the only thing I had eaten was that pastry. And that was the epiphany: Eating bad food causes problems. Or put this way: That pastry did not love me!

My journey into good food and healthy nutrition began at that moment. I started to listen to my body and learn everything I could about food and health. I gradually made the transition to plant-based eating, giving up dairy first, then chicken and meat, then eggs. The last thing to go was fish. Once I was 100 percent plant-based, I got into even better physical shape and felt amazing, physically, emotionally, and mentally, 24/7. The application of food as the best medicine we've got to advance human health became the focal point of my career.

Eventually, I had another epiphany, which led to the creation of this law: Love food that loves you back—that gives you better health and vitality. Processed foods, sugar, sweets, sodas, fast food, junk food, animal-based foods—these do not love you back. They make you sick. You may love these foods, but they do not reciprocate that love.

Think of this interaction like a relationship with another person. You may love that person, but if he or she doesn't love you back, it's an unhealthy relationship for you. You go around feeling sad, depressed, and rejected all the time. Why would you want to be with someone who doesn't love you back? You need to be with someone who reciprocates your love so you both can feel happy and fulfilled in your union.

In the same way, you want to eat and enjoy food you love—and that loves you back. This might require you to unlearn some food brainwashing—like that it's okay to eat your favorite meal of spaghetti and meatballs, as long as you work it off by exercising for two hours the next day. That's nonsense—and the reason millions of people have unhealthy relationships with food. They live to eat, all the while forgetting that we should be eating to live. That said, more thought should be going into what we put into our bodies and even more so into how our bodies react to it. I believe we can all love food, as long as we make the necessary adjustments to make sure it loves us back.

With this law in mind, I guarantee that you won't mind trading junk food for salads or cutting out sweets, aerated drinks, and simple carbohydrates. You'll love making a few healthy additions such as high-fiber oats and loads of fruits, including papaya, guava, and apple. It won't seem right that you should eat bacon over fruit. Instead of wolfing down three burgers, you'll go for a black bean burger and baked sweet potatoes. You'll start loving steamed broccoli with sea salt.

The reason this happens is because your taste buds will acclimate to change.

Having counseled innumerable clients on nutrition over a span of twenty years, I can say with confidence that our taste buds are persuadable little dudes, and they learn to love the foods they are with.

So, in as little as a couple of weeks, your tastes will adjust to plant foods, and those foods will become what you prefer and desire. The benefits of trading up nutritionally extend well beyond a few new selections of vegetables, fruits, whole grains, nuts, and seeds. Your taste buds become more sensitive to salt—and you will actually prefer less salty foods. The same goes for sugar. Ditto for chemical additives. When your diet is cleaned up and your taste buds have detoxed, all that food processing mischief will become, in a word, distasteful. You will love great food that loves you back.

ANOTHER HUGE PASSION OF MINE IS TO TEACH KIDS THIS LAW: that the best-tasting food is also great for our bodies. If kids reject "healthy" food out of hand because they assume it will taste bad, we are doing something wrong at home. It's an attitude our culture has drilled into us, too, and only culture can amend. Fortunately, the operative unit of culture is the family, so we can fix this issue one household at a time. I think you get the picture.

Stop and think about something: Food is the one and only construction material for the growing body of a child you love. Don't you want your kids to have the best nutrition possible? I do! Food choices exert a profound influence on the health of our children across their life spans. Let's help arm them with their best chances for ultimate wellness.

The health of people we love—friends, family, our children, ourselves—is a universal priority. How we all eat throughout our lives will meaningfully and quite predictably influence our health and longevity.

We know without a doubt that there is overwhelming evidence of a health benefit from diets placing greater emphasis on vegetables, whole grains, beans, lentils, nuts, seeds, and fruit. There is also a sense of urgency clearly issued from concerns about the health of the planet—that the environmental impact of meat-centric diets is unsustainable and untenable.

Our goal must be food we can continue to love, but that loves us, and the planet, back. I'm pleased to say there are new and easier ways to get there from here than ever before.

YOUR GREENPRINT
by Following Law #9

You will enjoy great health—and so will your children—for a lifetime. The Academy of Nutrition and Dietetics states that vegetarians and vegans enjoy a lower risk of death from heart disease, high blood cholesterol levels, high blood pressure, type 2 diabetes, obesity, and cancer than those who eat animal products.

MOVEMENT BEGETS MOVEMENT

My grandmother started
walking five miles a
day when she was sixty.
She's ninety-seven now,
and we don't know where
the heck she is.

—ELLEN DeGENERES

I OPENED THE FIRST CYCLING STUDIO in Miami in 1996. The first few weeks were slow going, with me as the only instructor. People would come through the door but were afraid they couldn't do the classes. Some were in their sixties, seventies, or even eighties. I encouraged them to give it a try; they could go at their own pace—no pressure. If they didn't like it, no big deal. But I urged them to at least take one small step—or few spins of the pedals.

Happily, most returned. Indoor cycling became a part of their everyday schedule. Some people started coming multiple times in a day. Within a month, every class was full. I noticed lots of new faces. There was a waiting list. People were lined up on their bikes, pumping pedals, standing to push harder and faster, dripping sweat, cranking up the resistance as the session progressed. These folks truly wanted healthier hearts, trimmer bellies, and more conscientious lifestyles.

It was at the end of that first month, after observing the progress my clients were making, that Law #10 came to me: "Movement begets movement." The more we move, the more energized we become. And the more energized we become, the better we feel. And the better we

> **" IF YOU WANT A HEALTHY BODY,**
> *YOU HAVE TO TREAT IT AS IF IT IS THE MOST PRECIOUS THING YOU OWN. BECAUSE IT IS.*

feel, the more we are able to accomplish. Motivation comes from the momentum you create by taking just one small step. The feelings of happiness and accomplishment that movement elicit tend to perpetuate themselves. It might seem tough and maybe even impossible in the beginning, but nothing is more effective at getting you to a second workout than the first.

I would go so far as to say, do something physical every day, even if it is as brief as walking around the block. Working out does not have to feel like work, be tedious, or have a specific structure (e.g., 20 minutes of jogging or 10 reps of such-and-such exercise) to be highly beneficial for health.

You see, exercise is a habit. The more rituals that get you into a comfort zone, the more likely you are to stick with them. Write exercise into your schedule and give yourself permission to take that time to pursue an activity you enjoy. You don't have to remind yourself to brush your teeth every day; it's a habit. Working out can become one, too. But if you do something often enough, chances are, it will soon feel automatic. Soon you'll love getting up to go to the gym or for a walk around the block. Yes, I said "love."

Commit to exercising every day, even if it's only for 15 minutes. Need extra motivation? Put reminders on your calendar or in a cell phone text message. Set an alarm for your exercise time.

Stay consistent about it, too. If you want to get paid every month, you've got to show up at your job. If you want a loving relationship, you have to work at it every day and communicate and share, and be there with love. If you want a healthy body, you have to treat it like it is the most precious thing you own. Because it is. It's not a good feeling to lose your health—ask anyone who is seriously ill, has an injury, or has simply been suffering with a cold for a few days.

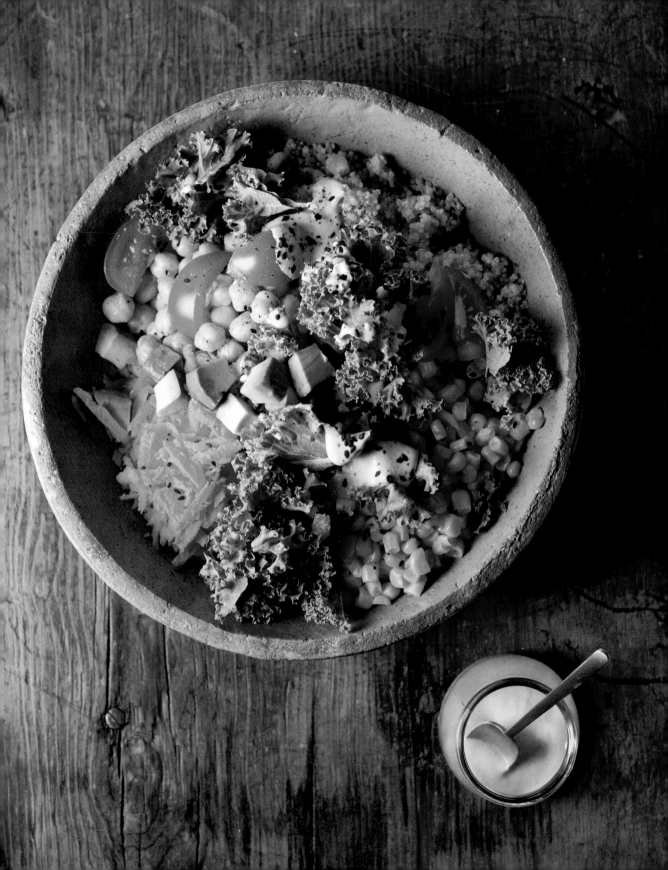

The sooner you realize that eating well and exercising are consistent efforts toward self-care, the easier it will be to do both.

Practice this new behavior over and over and over until you no longer have to think about it. It will be your life, not a quick-fix effort. It will be normal, a daily ritual, a habit, something so deeply rooted in you that you wouldn't dare skip it.

I start my day with a 3- to 5-mile run (some days more), and follow it up with some body-weight exercises (pull-ups, push-ups, burpees, dips, etc.). Some days I add some weights as well. I finish my workout with a great stretch and a few minutes of meditation. On the weekends, my family joins me for this! Yes, it sounds easy, and it can be, if you just put in a few decisions about what makes you feel your best.

Do it whether you're motivated to or not. We've all been there—you're on a great gym routine and then miss one day . . . then a second day, then before you know it, you haven't been to the gym in weeks, maybe even months. How do you push through when you don't feel motivated? You start moving. Take just one step. Maintain your momentum. The more you move, the more you improve.

Do exercises you enjoy, because if you're having fun, you're more likely to stick to it. If you're looking for permanence, you can't force yourself to do something. At the end of the day, it's all about engaging the body. If you aren't into tennis or despise running, don't do it! Find something you do like, and getting to the gym or workout class will feel much easier. Perhaps boot-camp-style training or yoga is more your thing. Whatever you enjoy, you won't see it as drudgery. Choosing your exercise routine is like choosing your career. You need to love your chosen exercise for a lifetime, so that you wake up excited that you get to go, rather than loathing the fact that you have to go.

At the same time, consider a few facts about exercise: To develop and sustain muscle mass and preserve strength as we age, it is imperative to continue to do some type of resistance training—weight training, for example—on a regular basis. This isn't just for bodybuilders or professional athletes, nor is it something you need to do just when you're young. The aging population, in particular, needs to understand that weight training is essential for preventing muscle atrophy. People think that if they're in their sixties, seventies, or eighties, they won't benefit from strength training, but nothing could be further from the truth. You start losing about 1 percent of your strength per year around age fifty, so you must remain engaged in a resistance-training routine or your muscles will weaken, which can make you more susceptible to injuries like broken bones.

Also, at the bare minimum, do some sort of stretching program one or two days a week, just so you can keep your range of motion. Even if that's all you're going to do, you still need to warm up and cool down. In order to warm up for an exercise or a good stretch, walk for 15 to 20 minutes so that you're on the edge of being out of breath. If the walk is going to be your exercise for the day, then try to walk at a moderate pace for at least a half hour. After a workout, I always recommend a good 10-minute slow- or moderate-paced walk to cool down before stretching. Your muscles have to be warm to reap the benefits of a good stretch. Think about a rubber band that's been in the freezer: If you try to stretch it, it's going to snap, but if you put it out in the hot sun, the rubber becomes more pliable and stretches easily. Your muscles react similarly.

Time your workouts according to your lifestyle. Exercise first thing in the morning to fit in with family life, for example. Consider getting up to exercise before your kids are awake. Exercise, shower, and feel energized for the day.

Alternatively, exercise on your way home from work—the next best action to exercising first thing in the morning. Take your gym bag with you so you avoid the temptation to stay at home when you swing by to get your things.

Have a big enough "why." Why do you want to work out? Whether your reasons are health-oriented or you just want to look better in a bathing suit, make sure your cause is solid enough to keep your routine

from fizzling. Exercise makes our bodies, our hearts, and our brains strong, and it helps us think and perform better. Other pluses are lower cholesterol levels, reduced risks for some cancers, and better overall attitude. Your fitness is the pillar that supports your plant-based diet so you can become fitter, slimmer, and resistant to illness.

Movement is naturally compelling for the human body. Getting back in touch with what feels good to your body can be a source of inspiration. So here's to play, new skills, new friends, or whatever else comes from your exercise commitment.

YOUR GREENPRINT
by Following Law #10

You will adopt one more lifestyle action—in addition to going plant-based—that promotes longevity. National Cancer Institute and Harvard researchers found that exercising 150 minutes a week makes you 31 percent less likely to die too early. Bump up your frequency to 450 minutes a week, and you have a 39 percent less chance of premature death.

TRASH MUST BE TAKEN OUT

> If we are creating
> ourselves all the time,
> then it is never too
> late to begin creating
> the bodies we want
> instead of the ones we
> mistakenly assume we
> are stuck with.
>
> —DEEPAK CHOPRA

"DETOX DIETS" ARE ALL THE RAGE, but what most people don't realize is that everyone detoxifies 24/7 without going on some strict regimen that might involve deprivation. Detoxification is a basic, natural part of being alive.

Our bodies detoxify naturally through the respiratory system, the digestive tract, the liver, the lymphatic system, the skin, and the urinary tract. You eat and drink what you need, and get rid of what you don't. You take in food and get rid of waste. You take in water and eliminate urine. You inhale oxygen and exhale carbon dioxide. For the most part, what you get rid of are toxins, useless waste products that can cause disease and damage cells if they linger in your system too long.

Detoxification is a two-phase process that involves enzymes that help break down food. In simple terms, phase 1 dislodges toxins and phase 2 eliminates them. Toxins that are dislodged but not eliminated from the body will be reabsorbed, causing unpleasant side effects such as fatigue, achiness, moodiness, or a general feeling of being unwell. The constant buildup of toxins not only harms your health and saps your energy but may also increase the risk of certain diseases, such as obesity and cancer, as well as conditions like arthritis, allergies, obesity, and many skin problems. In addition, a wide range of symptoms, including headaches, bad breath, fatigue, pains, coughs, chronic respiratory or sinus problems, gastrointestinal problems, and problems from immune weakness, can all be related to toxicity.

So what happens when you let your body naturally detoxify itself? My friend Emmet's experience answers this question in volumes—more than I could even explain. From the time he was a kid on up until age fifty, Emmet was a meat eater. As an adult, he had trouble keeping his cholesterol in a healthy range. And he battled his weight—which brought on a poor body image. Emmet didn't like who he saw in the mirror.

His wife urged him to try a 100 percent plant-based diet, but he was skeptical: "I had never been able to stay on any type of diet, ever. But I wanted to support my wife, who suggested that we follow Marco's advice."

At the end of day one, Emmet admitted to feeling hungry, but he was determined to keep going. After all, he had promised his wife.

Then came day three, and he woke up feeling "amazing."

"From that point forward, I fell in love with how I was feeling," he said.

Pounds started melting from his body. Emmet went shopping for new clothes for the first time in years.

As the weeks passed, he became fully and positively addicted to how he felt. Emmet did not want to turn back. Six months in, he had his annual physical, which included routine blood work. His doctor was astonished. Emmet's out-of-control cholesterol fell from 260 to 156. "What are you doing?" his doctor wanted to know.

"I'm a vegan!" Emmet proudly proclaimed.

Today he tells everyone, "I'm living healthier, longer."

As Emmet discovered, you have a lot to gain from strengthening your body's detoxification processes through plant-based living: more energy, vibrant health, a greater sense of well-being, joy in living, and inner peace, to name just a few benefits. Additionally, detoxification improves the way you look and think, eliminates allergies, reduces your weight, and helps erase signs of aging.

How can you support detoxification without subsisting on a special detox diet? Easy: a 100 percent plant-based diet, coupled with regular exercise. Both actions support the body's natural ability to rid itself of toxins.

PLANT DETOXIFIERS

The simple act of eating plant foods detoxifies your body naturally. These foods supply nutrients that specifically drive detoxification; animal-based foods do not. You have to eat plant foods in order to cleanse your body of toxins.

Plant-based foods also deliver antioxidants, which are helpful in ridding the body of free radicals created during detoxification. Toxins can morph into potentially harmful substances that can produce free radicals. So it's important to take in enough antioxidants to protect against tissue damage from these free radicals. Some of the best detoxifiers include:

GARLIC AND ONIONS // These and other vegetables in the allium family contain phytonutrients and sulfur that help move toxins out of your body.

LIVER-FRIENDLY FOODS // These include pears, oat bran, apples, legumes, artichokes, carrots, and dandelion. Certain herbs and spices, including turmeric, cinnamon, and cilantro, also support liver health.

FLAVONOID-RICH FOODS // These natural plant nutrients found in citrus fruits, berries, and green tea increase the activity of detoxification enzymes.

HIGH-FIBER FOODS // The digestive tract is integral to the body's detoxification process. This is where food is converted into energy and toxins are eliminated. Fiber in beans, whole grains, vegetables, fruits, and nuts helps reduce the absorption of toxins and sweeps them out through the digestive tract. Oats, apples, pears, strawberries, peas, and beans provide soluble fiber to soak up toxins in the intestine and escort them out of the body.

GREENS // Leafy vegetables—spinach, kale, watercress, and dandelion greens, to name a few—contain special components that support detoxification.

CRUCIFEROUS VEGETABLES // This family of vegetables, which includes cabbage, broccoli, kale, spinach, and Brussels sprouts, provides sulforaphane, which fights cancer by stimulating enzymes that detoxify cancer-causing substances. Cauliflower, cabbage, broccoli, and Brussels sprouts supply glucosinolates, which help the liver detoxify chemicals, including drugs and pollutants.

BEETS // These delicious vegetables are an excellent source of the phytonutrient betaine, which supports detoxification in the intestines, blood, and liver. Betaine also shields the body against the harmful effects of alcohol. Beets deliver protective antioxidants, too.

GLUTATHIONE-RICH VEGGIES // Asparagus, avocados, potatoes (with their skins on), raw spinach, okra, and walnuts are all notable sources of glutathione, a vital compound that helps remove fat-soluble toxins.

While you're switching to a plant-based diet, take out some other toxic trash, too. Translation? Cut out refined white sugar and flour, hydrogenated fats, and other processed foods.

THE SWEAT FACTOR

Water is a big driver of daily detoxification. In fact, drinking enough water helps flush out toxins through urine and sweat. Sweating in particular is a powerful health-builder. This natural, essential process is designed to help your body stay cool. But it offers superior detoxification benefits because it expels toxins from the body.

Although sweating as a form of detoxification has been kind of poo-pooed by modern medicine, it has been valued as a way to cleanse the body since ancient times. According to a review published in the *Journal of Environmental and Public Health*:

> *Sweating has long been perceived to promote health, not only accompanying exercise but also with heat. Worldwide traditions and customs include Roman baths, Aboriginal sweat lodges, Scandinavian saunas (dry heat; relative humidity from 40% to 60%), and Turkish baths (with steam).*

The review also highlighted the fact that toxins, including arsenic, cadmium, lead, and mercury, are eliminated in sweat and noted that sweating should be used therapeutically to rid the body of these toxic trace metals. That's amazing—work up a sweat, and out go harmful toxins from the body!

Sweating may help banish bisphenol-A (BPA) from your system. BPA is an "endocrine disrupter." This means it imitates or interferes with your body's hormones and throws your entire endocrine system out of whack. Although we're just now learning more about this toxin, it has long been known as a hormone disruptor. BPA was originally developed in the 1930s for its ability to mimic estrogen. It was a drug candidate for women with low estrogen as a result of menopause or other conditions, but was never marketed as a drug. Later, scientists discovered that when manipulated chemically, BPA forms a very resilient type of plastic known as polycarbonate. This launched BPA as a leading ingredient in consumer products, bringing this estrogen mimic, like a Trojan horse, into every home in everything from baby bottles to can linings. BPA then leeches into the food we eat and begins to wreak havoc.

The problem with a hormone disruptor like BPA is that the glands of your endocrine system and the hormones they send out are vital in calming your mood, promoting proper growth and development, regulating organ function, and controlling metabolism, as well as influencing sexual drive and reproduction. You don't want them disrupted!

HERE'S SOME FASCINATING NEWS:
Researchers have detected BPA in human sweat, sometimes even when it is not found in blood or urine testing. This means that sweating may be a powerful way to rid your body of this widespread toxin.

There are a number of ways you can get your body to sweat more. Nearly any type of intense activity will do the trick, although exercising outside in warm weather (or in a heated room, such as in a hot yoga class) will make even more sweat pour out. You can also stimulate sweating by using a sauna, either traditional or infrared. I like infrared saunas best because they expedite the detoxification process by heating your bodily tissues several inches deep. This boosts circulation and helps oxygenate your body. Traditional saunas heat the body from the outside in, like an oven. An infrared sauna heats up the body from the inside out, elevating your core temperature and stimulating a deeper, more cleansing sweat. In fact, studies have found that if you use an infrared sauna, your body will sweat out 20 percent more toxins, compared with only 3 percent more toxins that you'd sweat out normally if you use a traditional sauna.

A WORD OF ADVICE: Sweating, especially heavy perspiration, causes your body to lose water and electrolytes, so stay well hydrated if you've been sweating heavily, and replace your electrolytes naturally by drinking plenty of water and eating fruits and veggies. Also, if you do work up a sweat, please rinse off soon after in order to wash the toxins excreted with your sweat off your skin and down the drain.

The ideal take-out-the-trash program is eating organic, plant-based foods on a daily basis and maintaining an active lifestyle. It's easy, effortless, and motivating to know that these simple actions keep our body systems in good working order, around the clock, so that toxins are eliminated quickly.

YOUR GREENPRINT
by Following Law #11

You will immediately reduce your exposure to chemicals found in processed foods and animal-based foods. In a study from Emory University in Atlanta, researchers tested the urine of people who ate conventional and organic foods alternately for several days each. Concentrations of two widely used pesticides were not even detectable during the organic phase, but returned once conventional foods were reintroduced. Clearly, the ideal detoxification program is plant-based nutrition on a daily basis.

THE WORLD DOESN'T NEED US TO SURVIVE

WE NEED THE WORLD TO SURVIVE

> If slaughterhouses
> had glass walls,
> the whole world would
> be vegetarian.
>
> —LINDA McCARTNEY

WHEN I PLEDGED TO GO COMPLETELY PLANT-BASED, I started with a selfish desire to fuel my body and reduce my risk of disease, but then, almost instantly, I began thinking more about my impact on the earth and the treatment of animals.

I learned about animal welfare and the devastating effects of animal farming—things I had not thought about before. I knew eating animal products was making us unhealthy, and then I realized it was cruel, but I did not know that it was destroying our planet until I started reading more about the environmental effects of animal farming. The more I read, the more clearly I saw how plant-based eating could save our big wide world.

An Oxford University study published in the *Proceedings of the National Academy of Sciences* modeled the impact on our health globally between now and 2050 following four different diets: meat-heavy, meat-light, vegetarian, and vegan (basically plant-based eating). It concluded that if we ate less meat, 5 million deaths a year could be avoided by 2050; if we went vegetarian, the figure would be 7 million; and a shift to veganism would save 8 million lives a year. While it helps a lot to simply eat less meat, eating a plant-based diet free of all animal products is infinitely better for your body and for the world you live in.

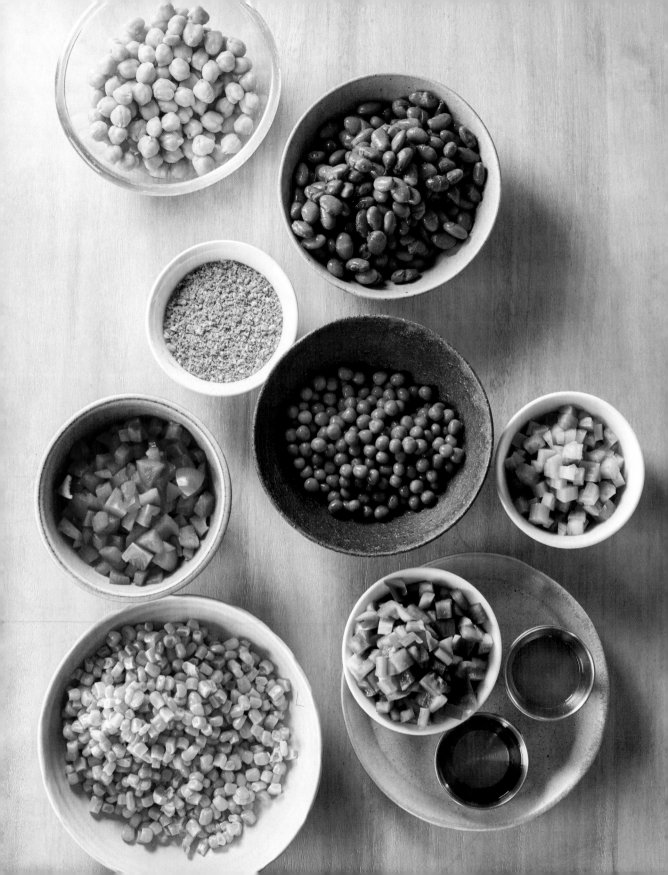

What we choose to eat has one of the biggest impacts on the environment of any human activity. Eating only plant foods is, I am now convinced, the best thing any individual can do to save our environment and our animals.

An Italian study reported in the *European Journal of Clinical Nutrition* in 2006 assessed the environmental influence of various dietary patterns combined with different food production systems. Researchers examined the effect of a typical week's eating on the planet. They found that plant-based diets are better for the environment than those based on meat. An organic vegan diet had the smallest environmental impact—the smallest greenprint. All non-vegetarian diets required significantly greater amounts of environmental resources, such as land and water. But the most damaging food was beef. Beef production required up to 100 calories of grain to produce 4 calories of meat. Mounting evidence suggests that every step of meat production, from feeding the animals to processing their meat, depletes resources and stresses an already fragile environment.

Animal farming is inflicting damage on a grand scale. It is a major contributor to climate change, discharging more greenhouse gases than all the cars, planes, and ships in the world put together. Raising animals to be killed for food releases more than 100 million tons of methane gas into the atmosphere each year, and cattle belch out huge volumes of it. Methane is a major contributor in global warming—it's twenty-three times more potent at trapping heat than carbon dioxide.

Carbon dioxide is another dangerous gas being unleashed into the environment due to human acts. The average car, if driven all day long, releases 3 kilograms of carbon dioxide, while the production of one hamburger releases 75 kilograms of carbon dioxide into the air—which means eating one hamburger causes about the same damage to the atmosphere as driving your car for *three-and-a-half weeks straight*.

According to the Environmental Defense Fund, if every American skipped one meal of chicken a week and substituted plant foods instead, the carbon dioxide savings would be equal to that of taking five hundred thousand cars off US roads. A little change goes a long way!

Cattle manure is a real problem, too. It's loaded with other pollutants like nitrous oxide (which is considered to be almost three hundred times as damaging to the climate as carbon dioxide) and ammonia (which contributes to acid rain that eats away at the landscape).

Livestock production also pollutes our water. Manure, antibiotics, and hormones seep into our water supply, along with chemicals from tanneries, fertilizers, and the pesticides used to spray feed crops.

According to the Center for Sustainability and the Global Environment at the University of Wisconsin, 40 percent of the earth's entire land surface is used for agriculture, and 70 percent of all agricultural land is used for farming animals. Farmland that could grow grain and other human food crops is also a casualty of the livestock industry. And one-third of the land suitable for growing crops globally is used to produce animal feed. When cattle are allowed to overgraze, the result is that soil erodes away, turning the land into desert.

Eating meat also creates food shortages. There would be more food available if more people went plant-based, because many crops are fed to farmed animals instead of to hungry people.

Many people who give up meat end up eating more fish, like I once did. However, eating fish isn't without its environmental problems. Overfishing is threatening the existence of many fish species. Fishing practices like bottom trawling cause untold damage to non-target species and destroy the fragile ecosystem of the seabed. It's been called underwater strip mining. Fish farming can pollute rivers and streams, harming the wild fish who live there. And according to the Worldwatch Institute, it takes 5 tons of wild-caught fish to feed 1 ton of farmed salmon. That's crazy.

I have also known for a long time that animal farming is a nasty business. Like everyone, I have seen those horrible pictures of the conditions endured by farm animals in factory farms—despite the fact that they are innocent, sentient beings subjected to a life of pain and suffering.

If you don't think so, here is a story. Some years ago in Montana, a Black Angus cow awaiting execution escaped a slaughterhouse by jumping a five-foot fence. She then dashed through the streets for hours, dodging police, animal control officers,

cars, trucks, even a train. Cornered near a river, the frightened animal leapt into its icy waters and made it across, until a tranquilizer gun brought her down. Her plight stole the hearts of the locals, who cheered her on and demanded her freedom. The cow was given a name, Molly, and allowed to live out her days on a nearby farm, grazing under open skies.

Most slaughterhouses in the United States kill more than a thousand Mollys a day—they're lined up, shot in the head, and often cut open and allowed to bleed out while still conscious, a cruel, terrifying end, full of bellowing. An estimated 1 million pigs die from crushing, freezing, dehydration, or disease on their way to slaughterhouses each year. If they even reach the slaughterhouse, they are rendered unconscious or suffocated with carbon dioxide, then dragged upside down using chains or ropes around their necks, until their throats are slashed so that they bleed out. Chickens are electrocuted before their heads are cut off with a rotating blade. Others are suffocated with carbon dioxide or their necks broken. Horrible, I know.

Even before slaughter, the animals are injected with hormones so they grow faster, add more bulk, or produce more milk in the case of dairy cows. All of those chemicals are transported into the bodies of the people who eat this meat. But our body systems cannot handle these chemicals, so, lying undigested, they can eventually lead to cancers and the weakening of our immune system. The meat and milk from these animals is also toxic and is rejected by the human biology.

It is interesting to note that physiologically our bodies are designed for eating vegetables and fruits. Our teeth are not pointed and our intestines are much longer than our bodies, very much like plant-eating animals. Carnivores have short intestines through which meat passes easily. But humans are different. Meat passes through our intestines much more slowly and is very heavy to digest, sometimes taking up to 72 hours. During this interval, most of it rots and ferments in our bodies. Plant foods, on the other hand, are digested within a few hours.

Ultimately, it's not our farming practices that need to change—it's our food choices. I believe that everyone in the developed world should consume a plant-based diet for health and for environmental reasons. We have to change.

Remember that the food you eat is connected to other living beings. This helps us make more compassionate choices. By taking a stance with our buying choices, we are helping to change our unsustainable food system and industry practices, because companies respond to demand. Just as little things matter in your personal relationships, little things matter in your relationship with the earth. Your choices create positive impacts that reverberate throughout the food system and inspire the people around you. When you change your diet to be more compassionate and sustainable, you become visible proof that changing our food habits is doable, healthy, and enjoyable.

YOUR GREENPRINT
by Following Law #12

To reiterate what I stated earlier: If you and your family go 100 percent plant-based, you can save two hundred animals a year, according to PETA. Not only that, but you can take a giant step toward preserving the planet. Leading authorities say that if every person ate the same diet (including animal-based foods) as the average American, we'd need 3.74 earths to sustain the world's population by 2050.

CHANGE STARTS WITH YOU

> You cannot get through a single day without having an impact on the world around you. What you do makes a difference, and you have to decide what kind of difference you want to make.
>
> **—JANE GOODALL**

IT'S A SCARY IRONY: We are dying way too young of heart disease and cancer while being told to cut down on fat and eat more plant foods. Yet at the same time, the agriculture and food industries are altering the content of those foods for the worse.

Consider the following chain of events: Enormous centralized farms grow single crops, relying on synthetic fertilizers for productivity and pesticides to wipe out pests. They have probably bought GMO seeds, because they produce tomatoes and carrots and fruit that look nice, resist disease, and can withstand being shipped halfway around the world—and thus a make a profit.

Sure, those fertilizers help the plants, but not the soil. The soil gets more degraded, while the pests become more resistant to pesticides. Thus, more pesticides must be applied, which in turn destroy the beneficial organisms in the soil. It's a vicious cycle.

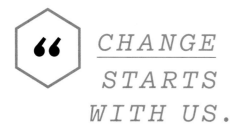

CHANGE STARTS WITH US.

All this occurs at the expense of our precious environment. According to a 2016 study published in *The International Journal of Education and Management Studies*: "The increased consumption of fertilizers has a negative effect on the environment. It may lead to water pollution, soil acidification, and trace mineral depletion and also degrades fertility of soil in the long term."

We have more food available today than ever before, but most of it isn't real food—it's chemicals, it's processed, it's pesticide-laden. It's food that can't be found in its natural form—and we've gotten it there!

Let's ask ourselves, *What are we going to do about it?* If, having read this far, you say, "I can't do anything about it," then we need to talk. Change starts with us. If we are to find the solutions to these environmental realities, we as responsible and caring citizens all have a part to play. Everything we do and consume as humans, from the way we live in our homes to the way we eat to how we operate in our daily lives, has an impact on the earth. It's important to examine our lifestyles to understand where we might be hurting the planet—and how we can stop.

Our food choices are the one single action that can provide better health for us and our planet. Unlike buying a new car or upgrading our homes, we will always have to eat, so diet is key in terms of change. The road to well-being starts with making informed decisions that will help you shop, cook, eat, and feel better.

It can be as simple as eating less or no meat. The production and processing of meat has the biggest eco-footprint of all consumption activities. In fact, meat and seafood are two of the most environmentally taxing food groups on your plate. The carbon footprint created by a meat eater is huge—3.3 tons per year per person. Over half that amount is due to meat (mostly red meat, but chicken and fish as well). Cutting out animal products, including dairy, can cut your footprint to less than half that amount, as well as free up valuable resources to grow food crops rather than food for livestock.

Eat fresh food, always—whole foods that come from close to the ground and are packed with nutrients. Focus on unprocessed whole grains, beans, fruits, and vegetables. These are more economical, better for your health, and less harmful to the environment.

Scale back your food budget. For every bit of food you don't need, that much less fossil fuel, pesticides, fertilizer, and water are required to produce it. At home, we like to plan many of our menus in advance, making shopping lists and sticking to them, so there's no impulse buying.

Also, look at how much food you waste in a day, a week, a month: the vegetable you forget at the bottom of the fridge, the apples you bought in bulk, or the bananas that have turned brown.

Greenprint your cooking methods: Save leftovers in glass containers rather than plastic containers or plastic bags, or make bulgur instead of rice more often because it cooks more quickly. Also, use energy-efficient cookware. Some materials, such as cast iron, retain heat better than others. Others, like copper pans, reach the cooking point more quickly with less energy.

Set your refrigerator between 37°F and 40°F to cool sufficiently without wasting electricity. Try "passive boiling": boiled water takes a long time to cool, so turn off the burner soon after the water comes to a boil, cover the pot, and let the residual heat finish cooking the food, fuel-free. Take the time to prepare your own food, rather than buying fast food; you will reap major health benefits in the long run. These are small lifestyle adjustments, but they have substantial and positive effects on our lives and on the earth.

Vote for change with your dollars, too. When enough consumers stop buying unhealthy foods, companies are forced to listen, and hopefully stop producing those foods. You have the power to stop this insanity. After all, you are "voting" at least three times a day.

This law is not meant to give anyone a guilt trip but to help all of us be more mindful of our actions and the consequences they have on our lives and on the earth. There are so many ways we can help.

Our planet is in trouble. And despite the fact that many things feel like they're beyond our control, we can help. We can consider our actions and how they impact the planet. We can buy, use, and discard responsibly. We can save our own lives and the lives of those who come after us. We just have to do it.

If plant-based eating can make us feel better every single day while also reducing or minimizing world hunger and global warming, why wouldn't we embrace it?

Everyone, no matter what their personal circumstances, has a responsibility. This is not just a "nice to do" action. It is a lifestyle decision that needs to be taken and implemented every day if each and every one of us is to reduce our effect on the planet.

Don't sit back and watch our beautiful planet and its people suffer—do something to make a difference, not just for one day, but for life.

YOUR GREENPRINT
by Following Law #13

You can reduce your carbon footprint enormously by avoiding animal products and processed foods and switching to vegetables and fruits. An individual who does that generates only 1.1 tons of carbon dioxide annually, compared with the 2.8 tons of carbon dioxide produced annually by a person who eats meat daily. Making minimal changes to your day can make a huge difference!

THE BEST STARTING POINT

IS TODAY

> We are what we
> repeatedly do.
> Excellence, then,
> is not an act
> but a habit.
>
> **—ARISTOTLE**

SO OFTEN WE SAY, "Tomorrow, I'll start that new diet," or "Next week, I'll put my heart and soul into getting in shape." But when we say these things, we are discounting today!

The truth is that the most important day you will ever experience is today. Making today your best, most productive, and healthiest day, no matter what your circumstances, is the key to your success as you begin your plant-based journey with me. So isn't it better to start now?

Of course! But where do you start?

First, decide that the next time you put food in your mouth is when you start your new lifestyle. Second, continue incorporating one or two healthy changes at a time on a gradual basis, and don't concentrate on what you're taking away.

// Have a bowl of oatmeal with fresh or dried fruit at breakfast.

// Add vegetables such as lettuce, tomato, cucumber, and sprouts to your sandwiches. Use spreads such as hummus or mashed avocado in place of mayonnaise.

// Pile on the veggies at restaurant salad bars.

// Keep cut-up vegetables and fruit in your refrigerator for easy snacking.

// Snack on nuts or seeds.

// Enjoy a veggie pizza made with vegan cheese.

// Stir-fry vegetables and mix them with brown rice or quinoa.

// Use "flax eggs" in baking. (See page 176 for instructions.)

// Add beans and vegetables to your stews and soups.

// Try a few vegan recipes.

HERE'S WHAT'S GOING TO HAPPEN: You will find that you enjoy plant foods and that they satisfy you, and you will start to lose your taste for some of the animal-based foods you used to eat. If you didn't like vegetables as a kid, understand that your taste buds change. Try them again. Maybe you have to prepare them differently. Some people don't like veggies that their moms used to overcook into mush, but find that they enjoy them in their raw, crispy form. Try them raw or steamed or roasted. If you still don't like a particular vegetable or fruit, no problem—set it aside and try another. There are so many others—enough to satisfy every taste.

Starting today, continuing tomorrow, and gaining momentum the next day will change your life. Simply put, you can't win if you don't begin.

BELIEVE YOU CAN CHANGE YOUR LIFE AND HEALTH

One of the great things about being human is that you possess the most amazing tool for personal change: your mind. Your mind can help you transform illness into health and failure into success—if you use it in the ways in which it was designed to be used. But do you? Most of us don't; we focus on the bad things in life that we don't want. We focus on sickness more than health, or on being fat more than being thin and fit. This tends to stack the odds against us. In most cases, focusing on what you don't want attracts more of it into your life and serves to demotivate you. It takes you into a mind-set that "Today isn't worth much, and tomorrow isn't looking good, either."

The key to success tomorrow is to begin thinking like a healthy, successful person today. And yes, successful people really do have a different mind-set. Unlike procrastinators and self-doubters, they have little or no negative self-talk going on in their heads, but when they do, they quickly stop it. Be aware of your self-talk and throw in a few positive messages of encouragement and praise.

YOU CAN RETRAIN YOUR SUBCONSCIOUS MIND BY TELLING IT WHAT TO BELIEVE. Repeat positive statements to yourself daily, in your mind or even out loud. Create your own statements, depending on in which area of your life you feel you need more self-confidence. Here's a sample:

I am a self-confident person with the ability to take care of myself.

I respect my body and health, so I will feed myself food that loves me back.

I control my food choices, and I make healthy selections.

Reprogram your mind and start building your self-confidence daily. You'll be amazed at the results!

BE CONSISTENT

Often it's only sheer consistency that pulls winners ahead of the pack. Some call successful people "lucky," but those successful people will tell you that more often than not, it was their consistency that put them in the right place at the right time, and allowed them to take advantage of whatever good luck happened along the way. The more consistent you are, the better your results will be. If you have a perfect diet on Monday and a perfect diet over the days that follow, you'll be ready to start over again the next Monday. Schedule many small wins into your day. These small wins are the fuel that will rev your success motor.

DON'T PUT IT OFF UNTIL TOMORROW

"I know I should make some changes" is something I hear so often, but when that statement fails to become a reality, I remember just how important this particular issue is. Have you ever wondered about the overweight person who says, "I need to lose weight," and then gorges on sugary food, or the smoker who says, "I know I should stop smoking," and then lights up another cigarette?

I can't claim to know exactly what these people are thinking, but I think what they say they know and what they believe are not the same thing. There are plenty of warnings out there about the health risks of an unhealthy lifestyle. But for some reason, for lots of people, knowing about risky behavior is not enough to get them to ditch their bad habits. I believe the main reason for this is that people don't think the risks apply to them. Consider the example of a hot stove. How long does it take you to learn that if you place your hand on a burner, you'll get burned? Not long. And once you've been burned, you won't do it again. Personal experience facilitates the progression from knowledge to belief, which results in a change in behavior.

You don't have to be burned to progress from knower to believer. All you might need to do is personalize the cause and effect of bad habits you've been warned about. Do a "fast-forward" in your mind to a time when the consequences of your current bad habits finally catch up with you. Make it really vivid. Feel the shortness of your breath, the lack of energy, the signs of getting old before your time, the creeping obesity. Then push Pause. Ask yourself how you'd react to that scary diagnosis if it were true.

If you're wishing you could go back and do things differently, then I urge you to change *today*. In fact, the earlier you begin, the better your life and health will be.

It is amazing how many people switch to a plant-based diet and start exercising when they believe it will help them get out of the mess they are in. By starting early, not only do you increase your odds of success, but you also have more options later in life. And for those of you who are pushing fifty or older, stop worrying. It's never too late to start making up for lost time and improve your health for the better.

In fact, this happened to a colleague of mine in the diet and fitness industry, Susan. She was middle-aged and had created many popular diets—maybe even some you've been on. For many years, Susan had high blood pressure and was on medications for it. Despite all her nutrition experience and following a basically good, albeit meat-based, diet, she had never, ever tried or considered a 100 percent plant-based diet. We sat down and discussed this. I laid out the research and told her miraculous stories of how plant-based eating reverses heart disease and increases longevity.

Susan shared with me that she had recently started a promising new relationship with a man who once had had open heart surgery. They were planning a life together, so Susan was game to go 100 percent with plant-based eating to help her and her new fiancé live happily ever after, and for a very long time.

Within about three days of eliminating animal-based foods from her diet, Susan's blood pressure went from an average of 140 over 90 to 118 over 75—which did not surprise me, because I see this all the time. Optimal, healthy blood pressure is 120 or less over 80 or less, according to the American Heart Association.

Susan was happy about that, but even happier about something else: the boundless energy she felt upon waking up in the morning. "For most of the past fifteen years, I've had to drag myself out of bed," she said. "Now I jump out of bed, and I can't wait to enjoy my day."

I was overjoyed to hear this, but again, I wasn't totally surprised. I tell people all the time about the energy they'll gain from plant-based eating, and Susan's experience is living proof. As for her fiancé, he dropped 12 pounds in the first ten days of plant-based eating, and feels physically stronger and more energetic than ever. He had a stress test and cardiology exam recently and passed both with flying colors!

Now committed to plant-based living for life, Susan is clearly a role model for those she loves. What you don't know yet is how good it will feel to be a role model for those who will come down this road behind you. When you start taking the steps today that ensure success tomorrow, you will inspire friends, family, and even strangers to do the same.

YOUR GREENPRINT
by Following Law #14

When you seize the day and become a vegan, in the first month, according to an article published in 2017 by Dr. Joel Kahn on his website, drjoelkahn.com, you will avoid the death of 33 animals, the use of 33,000 gallons of water for animal food production, the destruction of 900 square feet of forest, the creation of 600 pounds of CO_2, and the use of 1,200 pounds of grain to feed animals instead of starving communities.

PERFECTION CAN BE THE ENEMY OF PROGRESS

> A goal is not always
> meant to be reached;
> it often serves
> simply as something
> to aim at.
>
> **—BRUCE LEE**

AS A PERSONAL TRAINER, exercise physiologist, and athlete, I believe in leading by example. I got better at this after I realized I had to teach others to aim for progress, not perfection. True success is progress toward goals that matter to you.

Have you ever watched a movie featuring your favorite Hollywood star, whose body looks buff and amazing? Maybe you told yourself that you want to look like that—and woke up the next day ready to make it happen. But a few days later, you miss a workout, eat a cookie, or have a pizza and beer. You didn't follow your plan to the letter, so you throw your hands up in defeat.

A cookie won't make you gain 100 pounds. A doughnut won't make you morbidly obese. And a missed workout won't derail you from achieving your goals. Americans have this attitude that "if I can't do it 100 percent, it's pointless." That's self-defeating.

Say you enjoy chocolate. Maybe you're hooked on it. For you, a day without a chunk of the dark stuff just isn't complete. However, because you want to start a healthier diet, you've whittled your chocolate fixes down to only a few a week. That's a perfect example of progress, but not perfection. And it's a good thing: If dietary perfection is what you want, I hate to burst your bubble—disappointment and failure will follow. Both can lead to self-criticism, turning your mind against you.

Real life isn't perfect!

I'm not surprised that perfectionism is associated with numerous health problems, including higher rates of anxiety, depression, and eating disorders. But here's something scary: In a 2009 study reported in the *Journal of Health Psychology*, researchers looked into whether perfectionists were more likely to die prematurely than people without this personality trait. They followed 450 people over a period of six and a half years. At the end of the study, their findings demonstrated that risk of death was significantly greater for high scorers in perfectionism compared with low scorers. Also, risk of death was significantly lower for high scorers in conscientiousness (goal-oriented), extraversion (how outgoing and social a person is), and optimism. Lesson: Perfectionism is bad for your health!

Maybe you're wondering if going 100 percent plant-based has to mean going whole hog (or should I say "whole broccoli"?), replacing all animal-based foods immediately—or if it can be a flexible transition. Sure it can! You can make whatever dietary changes you feel compelled to, in whatever order and time frame makes sense to you, in order to get to the goal of 100 percent plant-based living.

Remember what I emphasized early on: You don't have to change every item in your diet. Start with one change, like meatless dinners, and build on that. Progress can be very incremental—and the revolutionary three-tier structure I outline in part 2 can help you on your journey. I always say that people want to jump from A to Z but they forget about B, C, D, and all the micro-steps in between. Set a goal of increasing the number of plant-based meals you eat over the next three weeks, for example. You might try a breakfast of raw oats with cold almond milk topped with raw walnuts, sunflower seeds, and fresh blueberries. Lunch may be a quinoa bowl with lentils, seeds, and sprouts, or a sweet potato with greens and beans. Dinner may be raw walnut tacos or a veggie curry or a raw veggie salad with tahini dressing.

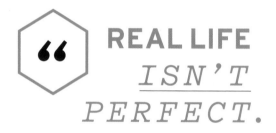

" REAL LIFE *ISN'T* PERFECT.

In the process, you'll discover that it's pretty easy to adopt a plant-based diet as you learn to love the foods that love you (Law #9). And you just have to keep thinking, *Progress, not perfection!*

One example of this is Soledad. In the beginning, she was a "perfection addict." She liked to compare her figure to stars and models who were picture-perfect—a habit that only led to greater dissatisfaction with her own body. She'd start a fitness program, then stop because she wound up feeling worse about herself. As a perfectionist, she ensured she'd never be satisfied with who she was.

When she began to work with me, Soledad decided that this time would be different. She'd focus on daily goals rather than perfection. If she had a bad day or missed a workout, she'd celebrate what she did right, not get down on herself for the deviations. When things went awry, she gave herself a pat on the back for the progress she'd already made. She focused on the advancement she had made as being just as important as the distance she had yet to go. Then she'd simply get back to her plan the next day or as soon as possible.

Little by little, Soledad began to see progress, which fueled even more progress. Before long, she was in the best shape of her life and even started competing in 5K runs. She achieved what she had never been able to before by simply doing what she had never done before: focusing on progress, not perfection.

Fitness and nutrition is not a game of "perfect." Trying to be perfect can keep you from trying new and untested methods for reaching your goals. Wanting perfection is fine, but expecting it is unrealistic. Strive for bold, resolute action in the direction of your goals, and plan to make course corrections as you go. Let your unrealistic expectations of perfection go, and your results will start to flow.

I firmly believe that tracking your progress is important. Set specific behavior goals and monitor your progress. For example, if your goal is to lose 20 pounds over the next few months, look at built-in progress-markers, such as eating clean each day, exercising several times during any given week, losing a few pounds weekly, and so forth.

Whenever I feel like I'm not doing something perfectly, I bring to mind a piece of advice I once got: Healthful living is about the journey, not the destination. At the same time, I remember there's an opportunity every day to do something good for myself.

YOUR GREENPRINT
by Following Law #15

You will make incremental but highly impactful progress. According to the Earth Day Network, these small changes over the course of a year can have big results:

// Eating one less beef burger a week is the equivalent of taking your car off the road for 320 miles.

// Skipping meat and cheese for one day a week is the equivalent of taking your car off the road for five weeks.

// Skipping steak once a week is the equivalent of taking your car off the road for nearly three months.

// And if the entire United States did not eat meat or cheese for just one day a week, it would have the same effect as not driving 91 billion miles—or taking 7.6 million cars off the road.

LISTEN TO YOUR BODY

Each patient carries his own doctor inside him.

—NORMAN COUSINS

JANE HAD NOT FELT WELL FOR YEARS, and she didn't know why. When her yearly physical found her blood pressure to be high, her doctor prescribed not one, but three antihypertensive drugs. She faithfully took all the medications her doctor recommended. But they weren't doing a very good job of keeping her healthy. In fact, she started feeling worse. Her blood pressure went down, but alarm bells started sounding. She was dealing with all sorts of side effects—fatigue, dizziness, headaches, dry cough, and memory problems—presumably from the medications.

This was her state of health when we met. Jane was convinced that conventional medicine had failed her. She was desperate to do something, because she understood the startling statistics: If you suffer from uncontrolled high blood pressure, your risk of having a heart attack is 300 percent higher than that of someone with normal blood pressure. Your risk of suffering a stroke is 700 percent higher. In addition, you're in the danger zone of developing kidney disease, blindness, or Alzheimer's disease.

Although physicians typically prescribe drugs as the first line of treatment for hypertension, the fact is that for the 80 percent of patients whose blood pressure is classified as mild to moderate, drugs aren't necessarily the best answer. In Jane's case, as with other hypertensive folks, there was another path to controlling her blood pressure: eating more plants and getting more exercise. In a landmark study called the Dietary Approaches to Stop Hypertension (DASH) trial, researchers found that a low-fat diet including fruits, vegetables, and foods low in saturated fat could lower blood pressure as effectively as drugs. Imagine the number of lives that could be saved with this one simple lifestyle change!

The diet I recommended to Jane was similar to the DASH diet, but with a greater emphasis on plant foods. In fact, I advised her to switch to a 100 percent whole-foods plant-based diet and work with her doctor along the way to check her symptoms and progress.

Jane began making some of these dietary changes. Within one week of starting a completely plant-based diet and daily 45-minute brisk walks, she was off two of the three hypertension medications because her blood pressure had dropped dramatically. A few months later, she went in for a checkup. Her cardiologist could not believe what he was witnessing: Her blood pressure was completely normalized and he proceeded to take her off the third drug. She continues to monitor her blood pressure on a regular basis and it remains within normal range. She continues to exercise and eats completely plant-based.

Jane is a good example of someone who practices Law #16, "Listen to your body." No one knows your body as well as you do, so don't ignore abnormal symptoms, even if they come from taking drugs that are meant to help you.

Our bodies are wonderfully designed with the most sophisticated built-in alarm system to alert us of potential damage before it gets worse. If a fire alarm goes off in a building or smoke detectors blare in your home, what do you do?

Well, you might find a way to turn the alarm off quickly with little to no concern about a potential fire. Or you might try to figure out what caused the alarm to go off and then address the issue.

Symptoms are like those alarms. They're your body's way of getting your attention so that you can respond to whatever is happening to you. Symptoms are important, but only if we address their underlying causes. The problem is, medicine tends to address only the symptoms resulting from the disease or its onset in the body, not the disease itself. Low energy? No problem—drink loads of caffeine. Can't sleep? No problem—here's a prescription drug for that. Losing your erection? Pop this little pill for that as well. Feeling down? Here's an antidepressant. You get the point. No disease or illness can be cured by patching the symptoms and not treating the underlying cause of the disease itself. Yet our society has built a massive multitrillion-dollar industry around silencing these alarms.

Sometimes, as individuals, we ignore these alarms altogether. I came across a story years ago that puts this issue into perspective, and I want to share it with you. Every year, a farmer planted and plowed around a large rock in his field. His experience with rocks over time had taught him that they are difficult obstacles to remove. Even after breaking several plows, he kept working around it. He got rather accustomed to this obstacle in his field.

One day, after losing yet another plow to the rock, he remembered all the problems it had caused him over the years. That's when he finally decided to take action. He placed a crowbar under the stone and began to lift it.

WARNING SIGNS

THAT SOMETHING MIGHT BE WRONG

How do we know when there's something really wrong with our health? Usually it's when we have major signs and symptoms. If you are experiencing symptoms like those listed here, seek medical attention.

1 UNINTENTIONAL WEIGHT LOSS

2 CHANGE IN A MOLE

3 SNORING

4 MORE FREQUENT TRIPS TO THE BATHROOM

5 INFLAMED GUMS

6 UNRELENTING FATIGUE

7 SEVERE PAIN ANYWHERE ON YOUR BODY

8 NAGGING COUGH

9 CHANGE IN BOWEL HABITS FOR NO OBVIOUS REASON

10 CHANGES IN HANDWRITING

11 INABILITY TO REMEMBER NAMES OF OBJECTS OR PEOPLE

12 UNEXPLAINED BLEEDING

13 IMPOTENCE

14 SHORTNESS OF BREATH

15 DEPRESSION OR ANXIETY THAT WON'T LIFT

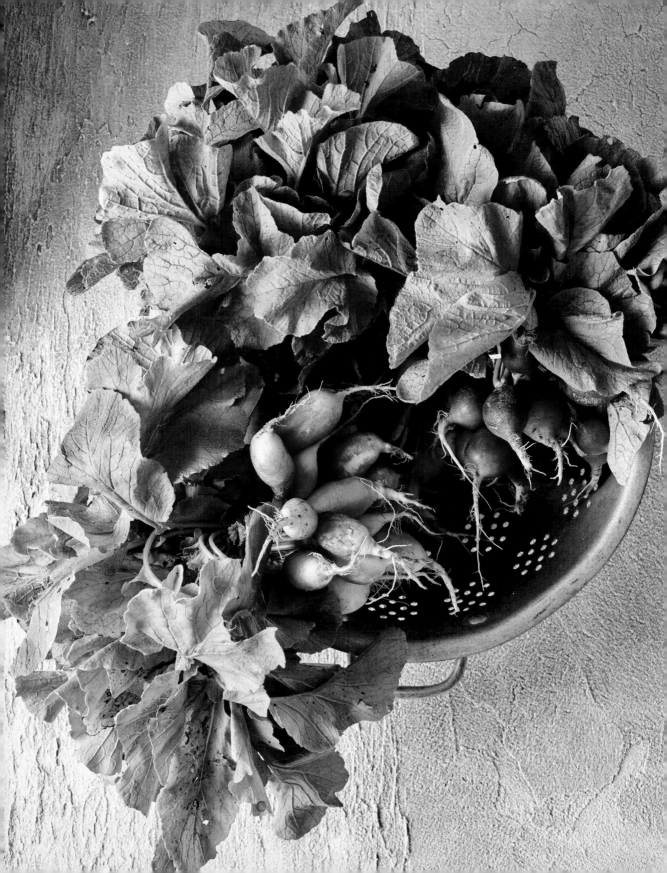

To his surprise, the rock was light. Once out of the ground, it could easily be broken with a sledgehammer.

Hauling the crushed pieces away, he remembered all the trouble the rock had caused him and how easy it would have been to get rid of it sooner. Once the rock was gone, his life's labor was much easier.

Like the farmer in the story, when we have stones of poor health causing us problems in our day-to-day lives, we often do not want to stop and take the time to deal with them right away. We take the easier path, instead of the "harder," correct path. We ignore or fail to recognize warning signs in ourselves. Like the farmer, we "plow" around them or tell ourselves we'll take care of them later. If the obstacle keeps cropping up over and over, we're better off taking the time to fix it right and be done with it. If we keep going around it time and time again, we had better stop and ask ourselves, *Is the cost to my health worth it?*

You have the power to decide what your experience is and isn't. Every minute of every day, you choose to pay attention to some things and ignore, overlook, or bury most other things. What you choose to focus on becomes part of your life, and the rest falls by the wayside. You may be ill, for example. You can spend most of your days ignoring the illness, or you can spend your days focusing on ways to improve your health by addressing what is causing the symptoms in the first place. By understanding what's really going on inside and doing something about it, you can achieve better emotional and physical health.

Our bodies are up front and honest.

They send us a series of wake-up calls. How you respond to these wake-up calls affects their power over the rest of your life.

So please, please, don't procrastinate. If you're putting off a medical checkup for your symptoms because you "don't have the time," look at it this way: A couple of visits to your doctor to figure out the source of your problem will prevent a whole lot more time in medical offices down the line. And in so many cases, lifestyle and habit changes work best. In the end, it really is about paying attention to your body and answering its calls. Listen to your body. It's trying to tell you something.

YOUR GREENPRINT
by Following Law #16

You harness the power of early detection, which means finding and diagnosing a disease earlier than you might have if you'd waited for symptoms to occur. That's why regular screenings and self-examinations are so important. The earlier the detection, the greater the chances of the disease or illness being cured. Take cancer, for example. Cancer authorities suggest that 80 percent of all cancers detected in their early stages can be cured, except for lung, pancreas, and glioblastoma multiforme (a fast-growing brain cancer), where only 50 to 60 percent can be cured.

FOCUS ON WHAT YOU CAN EAT,

NOT WHAT YOU CAN'T

> If I have the
> belief that I can
> do it, I shall
> surely acquire
> the capacity to
> do it even if I may
> not have it at the
> beginning.
>
> **—MAHATMA GANDHI**

WHEN YOU COMMIT TO CHANGING YOUR DIET, it's exciting at first. But often, you can fall into the trap of thinking about all the foods you can't or shouldn't have, that aren't healthy or safe to eat, and it's easy to feel discouraged. You may then develop an unhealthy attitude toward food. Food turns into an enemy, and every day becomes a battle. Instead of eating when you're truly hungry and to keep yourself in good health, you lapse into eating out of boredom, loneliness, or depression, or to comfort yourself. Everyone does this to a degree. Truthfully, food is your friend—so choose foods that make you feel amazing and complement your lifestyle.

The essence of this law is to change your attitude toward food from various negatives to positives. Don't feel guilty for eating something you like. (Remember, one cookie isn't going to make you fat!) Don't be stressed by all the foods you can't eat. Don't feel deprived. Here's what I suggest.

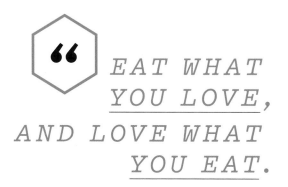

EAT WHAT YOU LOVE, AND LOVE WHAT YOU EAT.

EAT FOR NUTRITION

"To eat or not to eat" isn't the question. "To eat the veggie sandwich or the double cheeseburger and fries" is a better question. The choice may be between oatmeal and a jelly doughnut for breakfast—in which case, go for nutrition first. After you've had your plant protein, fruit, vegetables, whole grains, and lots of water, your blood sugar will be more stable and you won't be physiologically hungry. But don't choke down food you hate, even if it is nutritious. Find good alternatives. If you can't stand broccoli, eat a variety of other vegetables and fruit, and remember that it can take trying a new food multiple times before you acquire a taste for it. Additionally, studies have shown that most people *can* change their taste preferences, so give yourself some time to adjust to new flavors and textures.

CREATE VARIETY

Yes, I want you to eat more veggies. But you need to go beyond iceberg lettuce, celery, cucumbers, and carrots. It's easy to get into a rut by eating the same things over and over. A monotonous vegetable menu will quickly have you reaching for more fattening fare (I know, I've been there, too).

There is such a wide variety of healthy plant foods that can be added to your menu, so experiment a little. Some colorful suggestions from my family's kitchen include yellow and orange bell peppers, purple cabbage, spinach, beets, arugula, eggplant, blueberries, yellow squash, plums, and cherries.

Try new recipes, too. At my house on the weekends, my whole family gets together and comes up with new recipes. Raw vegan pie? We did it. Walnut tacos? Check. Spanish beans over sweet potatoes? Delicious, and now a family favorite.

As a kid, I was fortunate to be constantly exposed to different foods, an experience I've never forgotten and something I want my kids to experience as well. It left me with an enthusiasm, curiosity, and adventurous attitude toward food that I've carried with me over my life.

It helps, too, that my wife, Marilyn, is an incredible cook, so our four children have developed an appreciation for how good whole, plant-based foods can taste. My family's enthusiasm for discovering new foods to sample and new recipes to try is the foundation for a lot of wonderful things: good health, good habits, and good times together.

Let me add that your scale will thank you for filling your plate with a variety of plants. A six-month study led by Pennsylvania State University researchers showed that people who filled up on produce ate up to 511 fewer calories each day, on average, compared with those who consumed less fruit and veggies. So don't be afraid to try new foods and experiment with cooking.

GET THE PROCESSED STUFF OUT

It is really important to your health that you not eat processed foods—even if those foods are plant-based, like potato chips. When food is processed, the fiber is squeezed out so that you can consume more, faster, which means it's easier to overeat. Just because pasta started out as a plant does not mean that if you eat three bowls of it, you will lose weight. The opposite is true.

Do not feel bad about getting rid of all the unhealthy processed food cluttering up your kitchen. True plant-based eating is about giving yourself plenty to choose from instead of spending all day thinking about what you can't eat.

What kind of processed food is in your kitchen right now? Open your pantry and fridge doors and start reading labels.

AVOID ADDED SUGAR

This additive is everywhere and it's hard to avoid, even when you're aware of it. Added sugars come disguised under names like high-fructose corn syrup, corn sugar, glucose, fructose, sucrose, maltose, honey, molasses, treacle, fruit concentrate, dextrose . . . to complete this list of added sugars would take a long time. If you see any of those words on a label, don't buy that food! (For more information on different names for added sugar, check out the USDA's list at choosemyplate.gov/what-are-added-sugars.)

Common foods contain masses of sugar: tomato sauces, salad dressings, punches, peanut butter, pretzels, and lots of snack foods. Once I checked a loaf of sliced brown bread and saw that it contained 1.6 grams of added sugar per slice—that's almost $1/2$ teaspoon.

LOSE THE ARTIFICIAL SWEETENERS

Diet sodas, diet candies, diet anything. Eating plants is all about eating natural foods, not artificially created foods.

When reading labels, look for these names and brands of artificial sweeteners so you can avoid the foods that contain them:

Acesulfame Potassium: Sunnett, Sweet One

Aspartame: Nutrasweet, Equal

Saccharin: Sweet 'N Low, Sweet Twin, Sugar Twin

Sucralose: Splenda

TOSS THE PROCESSED WHITE FLOUR

Cookies, pancake mixes, cake mixes, white breads, cupcakes . . . get it all out. You don't need processed flours in your meals, because whole-grain flours are versatile and have all the nutrition the grain or plant grew with, plus the fiber and bran.

I love the great variety available to us in the flour category. If you're trying to limit carbs for weight loss or medical reasons, cook with nut flours such as almond flour. Nut flours are great swaps for regular flour in certain recipes. You can buy packaged nut flour, or easily grind your own: Place almonds, pecans, walnuts, or a combination of nuts in a blender, about ¼ cup at a time, and pulse to pulverize them (just make sure you stop before the nuts break down into nut butter). Nut flours add amazing flavor to baked goods. Plus, they're brimming with vitamin E, magnesium, fiber, and heart-healthy mono-unsaturated fats.

There are bean flours (such as soy, chickpea, and combination chickpea-fava bean flours), which have better texture and nutritional value than refined white flour. Healthy oil and a few other simple ingredients are all you need to add to these flours to create a tasty baked good in a jiffy. Chickpea flour is one of our family favorites. It has a unique nutritional profile and contains far more blood-sugar-regulating and help-you-feel-full fiber than most other flours. Chickpea flour is also a good flour substitute when people are allergic to nuts or grains.

You should never miss white flour or feel discouraged that you can't eat it. There are more flours you can eat than you ever thought possible!

DITCH THE DAIRY

Cheeses, cream, milk—I always tell my friends and clients to avoid these. There are many ways to enjoy your food without dairy. Use olive oil instead of butter, try cashew cheeses, and incorporate all sorts of nondairy milks, like almond, coconut, soy, hemp, oat, and rice milks—delicious.

FREE YOURSELF FROM MEAT

Processed meat, deli meat, hot dogs, chicken, beef, fish . . . Get all that stuff out of your house and out of your life for good.

Anything that shouldn't be there, bag it up, tie it up, and put it by the door. You can donate it, but if it's really bad for you, just throw it away. Know that in getting rid of it, you're doing something that's going to be bigger than you, because you've made a conscious effort to be healthier, to be better, to be smarter, and finally to be the best version of you.

MAKE YOUR DIET FIT YOUR LIFESTYLE

If you're constantly on the go, travel often for business, or work long hours, you may have to eat out often. That doesn't mean you can't eat healthy meals. When you really want something, you can make it happen no matter what. For example, when I'm traveling to a conference and I know the food they're serving isn't what's best for my body, I do my research. I'll try to find a hotel located near a shopping center that has a Whole Foods or other supermarket with a wide selection. After I arrive in town, I'll stop to pick up some healthy plant-based snacks for my room. I'll also research vegan restaurants in the city I'm visiting. Basically, I put myself in a position to succeed, and you can, too. The key is to know what you can eat and how to make wise choices when eating out.

The bottom line here is, emphasize what you *can* eat—and eat it often. Ask if a food is making you healthier. If so, you'll be eating more vitamins and minerals, less fat, and fewer additives than with unhealthy foods. Think of your eating plan like your budget for groceries—we all want to get more for less. The guidelines in part 2 can help you easily create healthy plant-based meals.

I once had a wonderful friend, Richard, who was a horticulturist. He would sing a familiar line from a Johnny Mercer song as he worked: *"Accentuate the positive, eliminate the negative. Latch on to the affirmative."*

What a wonderful philosophy! If we walk around complaining about all the things we can't have, then we'll likely never find true happiness and contentment. Alternatively, if we focus on what we can have, and how fortunate we are to be alive and live in this beautiful world, then it's much more likely that we'll find success and happiness.

Where food is concerned, when we focus on what we can't or shouldn't eat, we only crave it more. Focus on the foods that will help you achieve optimum health of the mind and body, and don't stress about what you shouldn't be eating. The cleaner you eat, the more you will start to crave plant-based foods. Eat what you love, and love what you eat.

YOUR GREENPRINT
by Following Law #17

This law is about focusing on the positives—what you *can* eat—in other words, being an optimist. When you're an optimist, good things happen to your health. Studies have found that people who describe themselves as being highly optimistic have lower risks of all-cause death and lower rates of death from cardiovascular causes than those with high levels of pessimism. The trait of optimism is an important determinant of how well and how long you'll live—so continue to focus on the cans rather than the can'ts.

PLANTS HAVE ALL THE POWER WE NEED

The world's
strongest animals
are plant eaters.
Gorillas, buffaloes,
elephants, and me.

—PATRIK BABOUMIAN,
strongman world record holder

THERE'S THIS TERRIBLE BUT somewhat comical misconception that
in order to be strong and powerful, we must eat meat. I often wonder
if those who believe this to be true ever think about the most powerful
creatures on earth and what they're eating. Elephants are the biggest
land animals, some of the most impressive giants on the planet, and
they're herbivorous. Rhinos, gorillas, pandas, giraffes, hippos, horses—
all plant eaters. Bison and cows, also plant eaters. And today, some of
the strongest, fastest, and most powerful athletes are also plant eaters.

I work with a lot of athletes, entertainers, and avid exercisers
who have switched to a plant-based diet for all the health and athletic
performance benefits it provides. As they make the transition, they
wonder if they need to eat meat to perform successfully. The answer
is a resounding no. As I've pointed out, there is plenty of protein in
a nutritionally balanced plant-based diet, and plant protein is much
better for muscle building than animal protein. When we exercise,
we create inflammation in our muscles. When you're in the recovery
process after exercise, your body wants to reduce that inflammation
so your muscles can properly repair themselves and grow. Eating meat
actually worsens inflammation. It's too taxing to your body. If you want

to truly build good, strong muscles, consume more plant-based foods, so you can minimize the inflammation in your body. The quicker you do that, the faster your recovery will be, and the quicker you can get into another workout.

Athletes and exercisers do need to ensure that they're getting a balanced amount of the nine essential amino acids that the body uses to build and repair muscle, among other things, but can't produce on its own (meaning you have to get them from the foods you eat). Amino acids are the building blocks of protein, and they're abundant in plant foods. The nine essential amino acids are:

1 // ISOLEUCINE: watercress, chard, sunflower seeds, spinach, kidney beans

2 // LEUCINE: alfalfa seeds, kidney beans, watercress, sunflower seeds

3 // LYSINE: watercress, walnuts, peas, lentils, brewer's yeast, almonds, chickpeas

4 // METHIONINE AND CYSTEINE: sesame seeds, seaweed, spirulina, Brazil nuts, oats

5 // PHENYLALANINE AND TYROSINE: sesame seeds, kidney beans, spinach, peanuts

6 // THREONINE: watercress, spinach, sesame seeds, sunflower seeds, kidney beans

7 // TRYPTOPHAN: spinach, turnip greens, broccoli rabe, asparagus, oat bran, kidney beans, watercress

8 // VALINE: mushrooms, snow peas, kidney beans, sunflower seeds, sesame seeds

9 // HISTIDINE: apples, beets, carrots, celery, cucumber, spinach

As you can see, many of the foods overlap under two or more amino acids, so it's not that difficult to ensure you are getting a good mix of aminos acids each day. You can also easily add some complete (containing all nine essential amino acids) vegan proteins like quinoa, buckwheat, hempseed, and chia seed.

Many athletes on a plant-based diet run into problems when they fail to recognize potential nutrient deficits *before* they become problematic. When you are planning out your plant-based diet, pay special attention to how much of the following nutrients you're consuming (which I discussed on pages 36 and 38):

// Vitamin D

// Vitamin B$_{12}$

// Zinc

// Iron

// Omega-3 fatty acids

The good news is that eating a good range of colorful veggies and fruits and incorporating a range of healthy fats into your diet will help take care of any potential deficits. Vegetables, fruits, legumes, nuts, and seeds contain an amazing array of vitamins, minerals, and fatty acids—we just need to make sure we are eating the right foods.

After converting to a plant-based diet, many athletes I know have experienced rather amazing benefits, including increased cardiovascular health, improved overall endurance, more energy, muscle growth, and reduced recovery time. Even so, there continues to be a lively debate over whether athletes should go plant-based. Well, not only do plant-based athletes continue to win medals and competitions, but science is stacking up on the side of cutting meat out of athletic diets.

In a study conducted at Arizona State University, vegetarian and vegan endurance athletes were found to have better cardiovascular fitness than—and be just as strong as—meat-eating athletes, perhaps in part because these diets are typically higher in healthy carbs, researchers noted. Ditching meat means finding plant replacements that offer more carbohydrates and more nutrients, and thus a more even delivery of energy throughout the day.

What about vegans and strength sports? Many weight trainers think a plant-based diet might be detrimental to their efforts; they fear they won't get enough protein. But we know this isn't true, since vegans get more than enough protein, and all the protein we require we can get from plants. Other weight trainers feel that a vegan diet enhances their training regimen by reducing fatigue and improving general health. Fortunately, researchers are starting to study vegan weightlifters and their nutritional needs. A study conducted in 2017, for example, revealed that a non-calorie-restricted plant-based diet burned body fat while preserving muscle—which is a goal of weight training, especially for competitive bodybuilders.

Contrary to what many believe, it really is possible to succeed on a plant-based diet in the highly intensive world of sports. When you train hard, you burn more energy and put stress on your body. You need to eat more as a result. Plant-based foods are an incredible source of nutrition for maximum workout power.

YOUR GREENPRINT
by Following Law #18

You'll pump up your body's supply of antioxidants, which can be notoriously low in athletes and exercisers. This happens because working out and training hard can increase oxygen consumption ten- to fifteenfold. Increased oxygen consumption leads to the formation of free radicals, renegade molecules that harm cells and destroy tissues. The best defense is a diet rich in antioxidants—which you get from eating plants.

A BEHAVIOR THAT IS REWARDED

WILL BE REPEATED

> Habit is a cable;
> we weave a thread each
> day, and at last we
> cannot break it.
>
> **—HORACE MANN**

NO ONE CAN ARGUE WITH the fact that humans are hard-wired to seek pleasure and avoid unpleasantness. As a college student studying psychology, I learned a law, often overlooked, that you must obey if you want to make lasting changes in your habits: A behavior that is rewarded will be repeated. If you ignore this, you will fail, as surely as if you tried to ignore the laws of gravity.

You will get nowhere trying to make yourself do things you hate to do. You will fail if you try to give up everything you like. You cannot forever impede your inherent tendency to do what feels good and quit the things you hate. To succeed in permanently changing your habits and yourself, to improve your health or solve your weight problem once and for all, you must find ways to enjoy what you like in ways that make you fit instead of fat or unhealthy. Believe me, there is a way. Every day, I train people how to do this.

When it comes to nutrition, you've got to identify foods you enjoy eating. Choking down a veggie burger and hating every bite is not going to help you change your food habits. Find plant-based foods you like to eat!

The same goes for exercise. You must find some type of physical activity you can live with, and eliminate every unpleasant, painful, or humiliating aspect of it. If a certain exercise class leaves you watching the clock on the wall, look for one that's fun and goes by fast. If your personal trainer is boring or unsympathetic, find one who is kind and inspiring.

Sometimes life gets in the way of living this law. Such was the case for Felicia. Years ago, she was following diets she didn't like, and as a result, she felt either miserable and sluggish while losing weight, or miserable and gaining it. She turned into a yo-yo dieter. This behavior ultimately wreaked havoc on her physical condition.

After she'd had enough of that punishment, she decided to try something different—plant-based eating. Felicia told me, "It pointed me to the right foods that energized me. It also taught me the best portion sizes and how to incorporate a more balanced mix of protein, healthy carbohydrates, and vegetables."

Felicia's new diet was rewarding, in terms of energy, a positive outlook, and consistent weight control. After switching to plant-based eating, she lost 19 pounds in the first twenty-two days!

In her free time, she loves running and is even training for a half marathon. She's up every morning at five a.m. to run, practice yoga, or cross-train.

Another reward of her lifestyle is greater mental clarity. "The food I was eating before was spiking my glycemic index," she said. "Now that I have a proper balance, I feel so much better. And I sleep so much better! I used to use melatonin to help me sleep, and I don't need it. I don't get sleepy in the afternoon. I sleep through the night and feel refreshed. I don't feel groggy. Plus, inflammation in my body has gone down a lot. My skin looks phenomenal."

Felicia's positive lifestyle changes have been well rewarded with loads of health benefits—which is why she is repeating all these behaviors, in keeping with this law.

The moral of her story—and of so many others—is that we've got to establish habits that reward us with positive outcomes so that we will repeat those habits. How exactly can we do that? I've got several strategies.

SET REALISTIC, DEFINITIVE GOALS // It's hard to focus on healthy habits if you don't have a goal—one that's measurable and realistic. If your goal is "be healthier" or "lose weight," without specifying parameters such as a normal blood sugar reading, a good blood pressure number, or a number of pounds, you'll have a hard time staying motivated, even if you start to see results. In the same vein, setting unrealistic goals will just set you up for disappointment.

By keeping your goals realistic and measurable, you can use your results to further motivate you toward your final goal. For example, if you want to eat more plant-based meals, your goal might be to eat at least one plant-based meal per day for a certain period of time then gradually increase that to two meals—which is what the Greenprint diet outlines for you. Or challenge yourself to the full forty-four-day Greenprint diet to enjoy the full benefits of a plant-based diet.

CUT BAD HABITS // Whether part of your ultimate goal or not, cutting bad habits is a good way to help you move toward a healthier lifestyle, which in turn will help you stay on track to maintain healthy habits. When you pare back or eliminate bad habits, whether it's smoking, drinking, unhealthy eating, or too much screen time, it will accelerate your results. Give yourself some time to identify the bad habits that are keeping you from starting your healthy habits.

PRIORITIZE // To achieve your resolutions, you need to put them in the forefront. This might mean moving some other priorities down the list, getting up a bit earlier, or reducing the time you spend on other, less important things. However, you can also help yourself make time by finding ways to save time—such as cooking large batches of healthy food, working out while the kids are at their activities, splitting up tasks to fit into your busy schedule, etc. Remember, this is about your health and well-being! Some people find that making a schedule helps—as long as you stick to it!

FIND FRIENDS // An important strategy for accomplishing your goals is to have support rather than go it alone. Finding a group with whom you can share your triumphs and tribulations can make all the difference. Even if it's just an online group, a Facebook group, or an email chain with friends and family, any type of communication can help you stay on track.

BRUSH OFF SETBACKS // Don't let small sidesteps derail your plans or guilt prevent you from moving forward. This isn't about perfection, it's about progression. The sooner you move on after a slip, the quicker you can get back to your goals. But before moving on, take a moment to analyze why you had the setback—whether it was stress, the difficulty of your goal, and so forth. This can help you prevent it from happening again.

If you happen to have a hiccup, forgive yourself and move on. Yes, it may take you a bit longer to reach your goal, but you will reach it. Tomorrow is a new day!

Above all, continue moving forward. Celebrate your successes (no matter how small) and brush defeat aside. In no time at all, your new habits will fall into place, and you'll feel the new you take shape.

You don't have to accept ill health, obesity, misery, and a shortened life span. You can change things and make your life better. You can be happy. And you do it by making your life more enjoyable, not less.

YOUR GREENPRINT
by Following Law #19

Targeting just one or two habits sets your course toward a healthier body and lifestyle. Let me use the example of Meatless Mondays, a movement founded in 2003 in association with the Johns Hopkins School of Public Health that promotes avoiding animal foods one day a week. Deciding to have a day free of eggs, dairy, and meat of all kinds is a positive step toward improved health, more awareness of the suffering of farmed animals, and relief for a world burdened with feeding more than 7 billion humans. The greenprint of just one day on a plant-based diet can also spur your transition to a 100 percent plant-based diet.

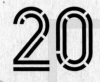

LAW

20

YOU CANNOT GIVE WHAT YOU

DO NOT HAVE

> Most of us spend too much time on what is urgent and not enough time on what is important.
>
> **—STEPHEN R. COVEY**

I TRAVEL FREQUENTLY FROM COAST TO COAST as the CEO for my company, 22 Days Nutrition. When I'm home in Miami, I spend as much time as I can with my family, even if I have to take red-eye flights from one place to another.

We all have demanding schedules. You, too, may often feel overwhelmed and overworked. Some days are so fast-paced, you may wonder if you'll ever be able to keep up!

On a recent flight home, I started paying more attention to an old familiar message from the flight attendant at the beginning of the flight: "In the event of an emergency, please put on your oxygen mask before assisting others."

I realized that if I can't breathe, I can't help anyone around me. It also hit me that securing my own oxygen mask was the most selfless and helpful thing I could do for everyone else.

I confess, it's a message I've often tuned out—take care of yourself first so you're able to help out in emergencies—yet it's one that can make a significant difference in our effectiveness. You can't take care of your family and friends, or do your best at work, if you're not taking care of yourself. And if you are physically or emotionally depleted, you won't have anything to give to others. So some of the changes you need to make may include taking better care of yourself and making time to unwind in whatever way you like.

But you know as well as I do that people do the opposite. They dart around like crazy, helping everyone else with their "oxygen masks"—errands, kids' activities, obligations, and more—and eventually run out of steam themselves, getting stressed, run-down, out of shape, and emotionally spent.

You can't give what you don't have. If you want to give more, serve more, contribute more, do more, create more, you have to be at your strongest and most vital. You must make *you* your first priority so you can be there when other people really need you.

What does putting on your own mask first look like? It's practically every law you've learned so far!

COMMIT TO LAW #1, "EAT MORE PLANTS."

Seriously, you wouldn't be reading this book if there wasn't something that bothered you about your diet, or if you didn't look or feel as good as you used to (or want to). A plant-based diet can help you with that, guaranteed. If you're starting to feel your mortality, then it's time to make a change that will help you live longer (and healthier). It's hard to believe, but other than saving the lives of animals, a vegan lifestyle can save the lives of human beings—specifically, yours. Studies have shown that people with a plant-based diet live four to seven years longer than others, particularly if their lifestyle includes a limited intake of alcohol and tobacco products. Cutting out meat and increasing your intake of fruits and vegetables can dramatically cut your risk of chronic disease.

DRINK WATER THROUGHOUT THE DAY

By staying hydrated, you'll be taking care of your most basic needs first. Also, make sure to eat enough to ensure your blood sugar isn't crashing. Have healthy snacks around, especially when you are ruled by your or your children's busy schedules.

MOVE YOUR BODY FOR AT LEAST 30 MINUTES FOUR TIMES A WEEK

Do something you love, whether it's strength training, indoor cycling, yoga, or walking. Just get out and move.

TAKE TIME OFF FROM THE DIGITAL STUFF IN YOUR LIFE

While computers, television, laptops, smartphones, and social media may feel relaxing and allow you to turn "off," try to find a screenless activity to truly take time for yourself.

ENACT EVEN THE SMALLEST RITUALS OF SELF-CARE

This might mean taking a warm bath, cleansing and moisturizing your face, going for a massage, listening to relaxing music with a cup of tea, or journaling what you are grateful for.

GET A GOOD NIGHT'S SLEEP TO HELP YOUR BODY PUSH ITS RESET BUTTON

If you want the nutrition you give your body to be able to help you heal and repair your muscles and organs after you work out, you're going to need some rest. Adequate sleep is fundamental for good health; it helps you regenerate and release stress. It's also vital for feeling energized during the day. People who don't sleep enough make poor choices, are more irritable, and snack more.

BLOCK OUT TIME FOR YOU

Schedule some uninterrupted free time for yourself just as you would set aside time for a dentist's appointment or a conference call. Make time for exercise, fun, massages, shopping, socializing, relaxation, and recreation, among other activities. Be kind, gentle, and patient with yourself, and pace yourself. Never feel that you're being selfish; you can't give the best of yourself if you're not your best self!

LEARN HOW TO TAKE CARE OF YOURSELF EMOTIONALLY

Most people don't even think about taking care of their emotional health. They are too busy working, shopping, and wishing for more. And still, with all the striving for more, there is an emptiness that comes from such a mind-set.

That emptiness can be filled with love. Human beings are not built to survive alone. We are social beings who thrive with companionship, friendship, family, and pets. Which brings me to a very important part of being successful and emotionally fulfilled at everything you do: your support systems. Your parents and children and sisters and brothers. Your friends. The people who care about you. The pets that show you unconditional love. The healthier you are, the more readily you can take care of them, and the easier it is for them to support you—and the more enjoyable everything becomes.

In my work with clients, I've seen how each of these "oxygen masks" can help ease stress or offer just enough space to catch one's breath. Those who live this law reap the benefits of greater health, peace of mind, strong results, and better relationships.

So put your own mask on first, and you'll have everything you need to be healthy and successful, and to support everything and everyone else in your world.

YOUR GREENPRINT
by Following Law #20

Prioritizing your health by choosing plant-based eating keeps you healthy and strong for those you love, because plant-based eating protects the body against chronic diseases.

BRING MINDFULNESS TO EATING

In today's rush we all
think too much, seek
too much, want too much,
and forget about the
joy of just being.

—ECKHART TOLLE

WHAT IS YOUR HABIT AROUND EATING? Do you eat standing at the
counter with one hand in the fridge and the other in your mouth? Do
you eat in front of the TV or while reading or on the phone? Do you eat
when you're not hungry? Do you wolf down food so fast you can't even
remember what you just ate?

If you're like a lot of people, the answer to these questions is yes.
In today's world, people barely pay attention to the act of eating as
they grab food from packages, straight from the fridge, at drive-thrus,
and from vending machines. The consequence of this is that we've
become increasingly out of touch with our body's sense of hunger and
fullness, as well as with our enjoyment of food.

Enter the practice of mindful eating. It not only focuses on
what foods we eat, but on how our bodies feel when eating them. It is
about slowing down and taking pleasure in food. For me, it means not
scarfing down my meals or eating what will satisfy me in the moment
with no regard for where it came from, what is in it, or how it will affect
my body. I allow food that comes out of the ground to be the center
of a sensory adventure. Mindful eating encompasses how the food is
prepared, the environment in which it is served, the people with whom I
eat, and the attitude I bring to the table.

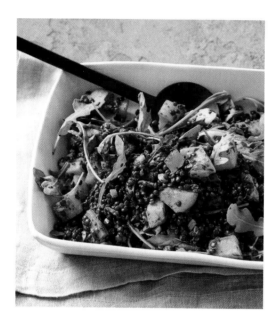

Because I enjoy cooking and creating new plant-based recipes, I bring mindfulness to this process, too. One of the recipes I recently created called for five different vegetables. Really focusing and taking my time with the prep work, I carefully washed, peeled, and sliced them while attuning myself to the steady rhythm of my paring knife, relishing the sound it made against the cutting board.

I intently listened to the sounds the veggies made as they simmered in a pan on the stovetop. Deeply inhaling their aromas not only made me feel like a good cook but also made me feel just plain good. There is enormous vitality in mindful cooking!

When I talk to clients who want to lose weight on a plant-based program, I encourage them to follow this law. Eating mindfully can help you reach and maintain a healthy weight. After all, if you're eating mindfully, you won't eat a whole bag of Cheetos!

In a Cleveland Clinic study, researchers enrolled volunteers in a 15-week online program that used mindful eating to help alter their eating habits. The dieters who were assigned to a mindful eating group used strategies such as planning meal and snack times, paying attention to how food tasted, and eating just one or two bites of higher-calorie foods. When the study concluded, the mindful dieters averaged a weight loss of about 5 pounds, while the folks who did not practice mindful eating had lost only about $1/2$ pound on average.

One of the most impressive benefits is in the treatment of obesity, which, of course, is one of the most pressing health issues in the United States. A literature review published in 2014 in *Obesity Reviews* made the point that weight problems are often associated with binge eating, emotional overeating, and eating in response to food

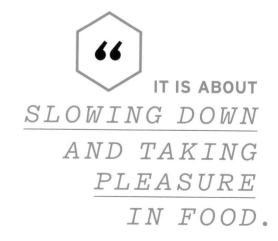

IT IS ABOUT
SLOWING DOWN
AND TAKING
PLEASURE
IN FOOD.

MINDFUL MANTRAS

FOR MEALTIME

Recent studies suggest that people who practice meditation may live longer and look younger as they age. Make mealtime a meditative experience by choosing and repeating mantras that resonate with you. Here are some examples:

When I prepare fresh, healthy meals instead of processed food, it is an act of love toward myself and those I cook for.

I choose foods well so that I can feel well.

I take in healthy nutrition, and I am nourished.

Fresh whole plant foods are gifts, and I eat them gratefully.

I enjoy the health and energy in my body, and I nourish it each day.

Nutrition is vital for everything I do, so I make it an important part of my life and set aside time to eat well.

When I eat plants, I feel energized and abundant.

I honor my health by preparing my meals with gratitude, mindfulness, and a loving heart.

I eat only what I need, and I stop before I feel uncomfortable or overly full.

I am grateful for how much the earth gives to me and how much I can give back.

When I eat fresh whole plant foods, I feel connected to the earth and the hands that grew the food, and I am grateful.

My body is one of the most precious gifts I will ever receive, an extraordinary creation that I cherish and use fully.

cravings. The article went on to demonstrate that mindful eating reduces the severity and frequency of these problematic eating behaviors—that people with these issues who practice mindful eating can lose weight and keep it off.

Mindful eating can have some real benefits if you are trying to lose weight, but in what other ways can you benefit from mindful eating?

Mindfulness offers an extraordinary and powerful ripple effect on how you look at the world, bringing happiness and calmness, raising your self-esteem, and making you feel like life is going to be okay. We all need that. If you value your physical and mental health, it makes sense to establish mindful eating and cooking patterns.

So what does true mindful eating entail?

To start following this law, ask yourself the following questions:

WHY DO I EAT? Consider your mood and how it may upset your eating habits. Be aware of when you eat for reasons other than hunger, such as stress, sadness, boredom, or fatigue.

HOW DO I EAT? Think about habits that may distract you while eating, such as watching television, surfing the internet, or driving. These habits move your attention from your eating experience and can cause you to overeat.

HOW MUCH DO I EAT? Quantity can be determined by your eating environment, your ability to sense how full you are, and your habits.

Then get mindful at the table!

CHECK YOUR HUNGER AND FULLNESS

How often do you finish a meal with your gut full to bursting and your pants too tight at the waist, wishing you could take a nap? That feeling of overfullness is one of the things that can make people gain weight. A feeling of "just enough" is just what you're looking for.

Before taking your first bite of food, do a hunger/fullness check: Gauge your level of hunger on a scale from 1 to 10. For example, 10 means you are completely full and can't take another bite, and 1 means you are ravenous. Avoid waiting to eat until you are at a 1 or 2, but continue gauging your hunger/fullness throughout the meal and be sure to stop eating before you get to a 9 or 10.

Twenty minutes after a meal, when your body has had a chance to begin digesting your food and processing your hunger level, you're perfect. Our bodies are very sophisticated, amazing machines, but in this technological world of immediate, at-your-fingertips gratification, we need to be patient. If you're not patient and you take too many bites so you can feel satisfied immediately, you'll regret it. You won't feel well, your stomach will hurt, and you'll feel lethargic—all of which are the opposite of your intentions when you sit down for a meal.

Really, your food should make you feel like you're ready to get up and go! Remember to practice this law if you really want to enjoy your food and nourish yourself.

ELIMINATE UNNECESSARY DISTRACTIONS

I'm talking about cell phones, television, and so forth. Stay present and focused as you unhurriedly enjoy your food. That way, you become more mindful of your senses and eat only what you need to satisfy yourself.

CREATE A PEACEFUL EATING ENVIRONMENT

See what you can do to get into the moment of food. Sit down when you eat. Eat at the dining table. Use a real plate and a real napkin. Light some candles. Put on some quiet music. Find a cool, quiet spot to sit and relax, or enjoy a meal with your best friends. These actions help cultivate a pleasurable atmosphere in which to enjoy your meal and feel good afterward.

BE CONSCIOUS OF YOUR FOOD WHILE YOU EAT

How does the food taste? Is it crispy, chewy, sour, sweet? You will soon start to notice and enjoy smells, textures, and flavors you've never experienced, bringing joy into every bite.

BE MINDFUL OF TRIGGERS

If you're like most people, there will be some situations that trigger your desires. Who doesn't want candy at the candy shop, cookies at the bakery, ice cream cones at the ice cream shop? Mindfulness in these situations helps us stay aware of challenges. So if you find yourself in a situation that tests your willpower, analyze it and prepare yourself for the next one, because the next situation is coming, and it's coming quickly. Stay mindful and aware. Put yourself in situations where you will succeed.

With practice, this law frees you of reactive, habitual patterns of thinking, feeling, and acting. Mindfulness promotes balance, choice, and wisdom. With mindful eating, you can listen to your body and know what you need.

> ## YOUR GREENPRINT
> *by Following Law #21*
>
> A more thoughtful way of eating can bring you better health and more happiness. In fact, studies of mindful eating show that it can alter food behaviors like emotional and stress eating that are associated with poor food choices and weight gain (and can lower levels of depression and anxiety).

PRACTICE KAIZEN

> A journey of a
> thousand miles begins
> with a single step.
>
> **—LAO-TZU**

CHANGE IS HARD, OR IS IT?

You probably have health and fitness goals you'd like to achieve. You know, things like losing some weight, quitting smoking, or becoming more active. But too often, you've given up because you think the goals are too far out of reach or the obstacles insurmountable, or because you try to change too much at one time. The key to meeting your goals is to break them down into small steps.

You can do this by focusing on *kaizen* (pronounced *kai-zen*). *Kaizen*, Japanese for "good change," is a Japanese concept for small, incremental improvements. Interestingly, it's the method behind the manufacturing and business processes that brought Japan back from near devastation at the end of World War II to become an economic powerhouse. Today, it has found a home in big business. In manufacturing and engineering, *kaizen* is used to identify the places in which mistakes are made or where systems could run more smoothly. It encourages us to look more closely and adopt tiny, effective shifts that can have huge ripple effects. Though it may sound arcane, *kaizen* can be a valuable tool that anyone can use to improve their health and fitness.

Kaizen is a powerful method for forming positive habits. For many of us, big goals like losing weight trigger fear. This fear of change is rooted in our brain's physiology—we are actually wired to resist change. But by taking small steps, you can override your programming so that you form new connections between brain cells and your resistance to

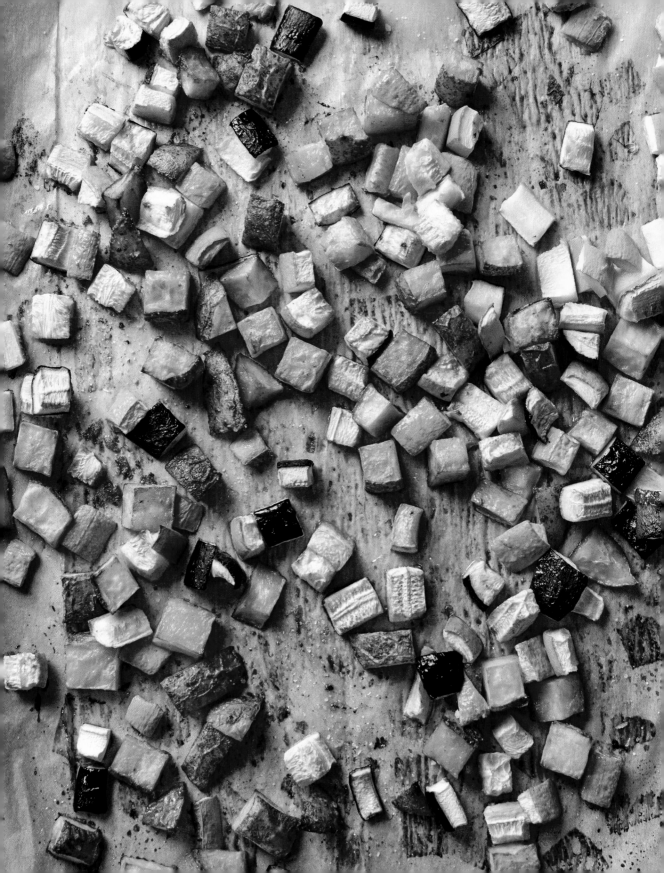

change begins to weaken. Your brain then enthusiastically takes over the process of change, and you move rapidly toward your goal.

In *kaizen,* you start by identifying something you want to change, then break it down into steps so small they appear to require little or no effort: lose 1 pound, eat one additional serving of veggies each day, drink one extra glass of water every day, walk for 10 minutes. These actions put you in the right frame of mind, and your brain and body then begin to develop the new habit. This is like the tortoise-and-hare example of transformation: Small, deliberate steps can usually help you achieve your goal faster than if you sprint toward the finish and get distracted or lose steam along the way.

Remember when you learned how to drive a car? You didn't just hop in the driver's seat, listen to someone explain how to drive, and then hit the highway. Not at all. You took small steps—turn on the ignition, put the car in gear, step on the gas—and you practiced all these little steps in a parking lot. You had to think continuously about what you were doing. A lot was happening in your conscious mind. It was stressful and overwhelming in the beginning. All you could do was focus on driving—the lights, signs, and other drivers.

You tried and tried, and practiced those steps some more, and eventually you could drive. Now when you get in the car, you barely give it any thought. It is nestled within your subconscious mind.

That is the habit-creation process. When something becomes a habit, the brain does not need to pay close attention as it carries out that action. Only the neurons at the beginning and the end have to fire, and in the meantime, you can think about what you have to pick up from the grocery store or what phone calls you need to make when you get to work.

The same process can work in your life when you change your diet to a plant-based one. Eating plants begins as a choice, but with small changes repeated over time, it becomes a habit—a habit that maximizes your energy and health, keeps you lean, and cuts your risk of serious diseases.

As you begin, remember that you are reprogramming your brain, and that it takes time for new mental pathways and connections to form. So choose an action, and perform it repeatedly over the course of several days or weeks. In other words, stay at it.

A few years ago, I heard a story that instantly changed my understanding of *kaizen.* The story goes that there was a man who had a very, very big oak tree in his back garden. He wanted to cut down the tree. He could not afford to hire a tree-felling service, however, nor did he want to buy a chainsaw for only this one tree. He decided to cut down the tree himself. With an ax!

Every morning, he went into his yard with his ax and swung at the tree five times. *Chop . . . chop . . . chop . . . chop . . . chop . . .* Five strokes only. Every day. Without fail. You can guess the ending by now! Within no time, he had cut down the tree. This story teaches us that there is real strength and value in doing something persistently and consistently over a period of time—and in tiny, patient steps.

Kaizen has been put into practice in many aspects of business and life—including eating.

HERE'S HOW THE KAIZEN APPROACH TO EATING CAN WORK.

ANALYZE

Before you take action, look at your current lifestyle. Keeping a food journal for a week is an excellent place to begin. At the end of seven days, you can step back and take a look. Is there one change you can make to your diet and exercise habits for the coming week? That one change can put you on the path to total wellness, one step at a time.

ONE CHANGE

Dumping your current diet for one that's brand-new and a complete change from what you're used to can be too much—so why not try something simpler? Here are some ideas:

// Drop one unhealthy food and replace it with one healthy food, like swapping out refined pasta for brown rice or quinoa.

// Use almond milk or another nondairy alternative instead of dairy milk.

// Try eating at least two vegetables with dinner.

// Try Meatless Mondays for a month and see how you feel—odds are that you'll notice you feel better and have more energy, and you may even consider extending your plant-based diet to a few more days a week.

// Grill, steam, or bake foods instead of frying them.

// Use spices instead of salt. Or use half the amount of salt.

// Have fruit for dessert; try baked apples, pears, or a fruit salad.

Do one of these for one week, and then replace it with something else. Within a few weeks, you'll start to notice how you feel: healthier and happier, which will help encourage you to keep going.

KEEP A TREAT

When you cut out everything that's unhealthy (or that you consider hands-off), eventually you'll cave and feel guilty. Instead, build a treat into your diet plan so it's part of your routine, rather than a departure from it. This could be a weekly glass of wine or dessert, or perhaps a monthly trip to your favorite restaurant. You will probably find that over time, your desire for those treats changes as your palate and lifestyle change.

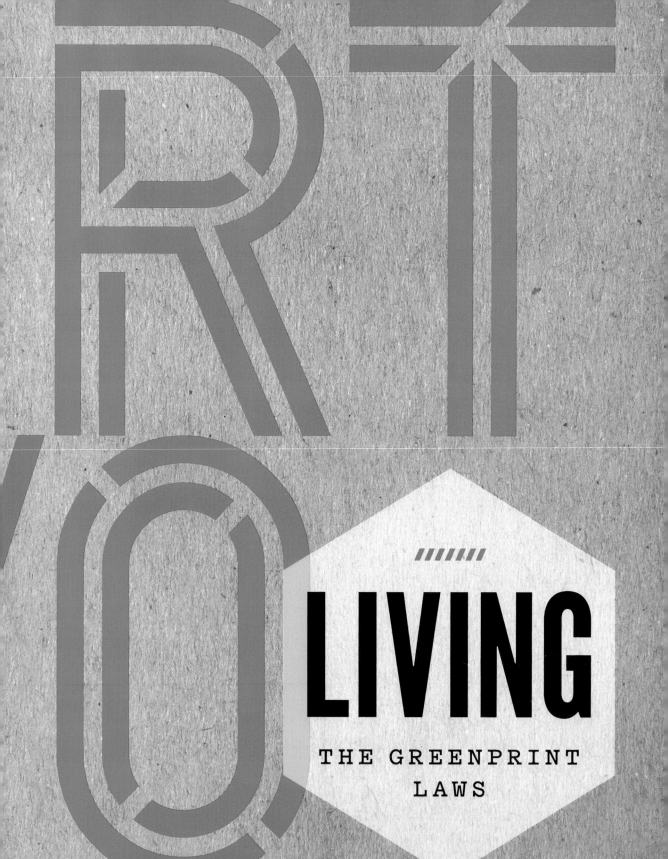

LIVING

THE GREENPRINT
LAWS

THE THREE

TRANSITIONAL TIERS

START SLOWLY

If you begin with lofty goals, odds are you're going to find it difficult to follow your plan and feel terrible if you're be unable to stick to your goals. If you start small, then you'll find it easier to adhere to your plan and keep going. For example, rather than trying to work out five days per week, start with two. If you haven't exercised in a long while, perhaps walking a few days a week is a good place to start.

KAIZEN YOUR WAY TO A HEALTHIER PLANET

The *kaizen* path encourages us to acknowledge that we can take small steps toward a healthier planet, too, like buying locally grown asparagus at a farmers' market in our town instead of supermarket asparagus flown in from Chile. When shopping, choose products with the least packaging or with the most recyclable packaging. Once you start taking small steps, they become integral parts of your lifestyle, and you will not think twice about them. Once you experience a few small wins, taking bigger steps becomes easier. Those, too, will become part of your lifestyle. Eventually, this is what always changes the world.

With *kaizen*, you can raise your standards of health and fitness, start and complete major tasks, follow a diet successfully, triple your energy level, and build your character to achieve a more fulfilling life. While your individual efforts are small steps, they add up. Even small steps taken consistently toward your goal move you in the right direction.

YOUR GREENPRINT
by Following Law #22

Simple steps through *kaizen* can make a big impact on health. Despite the daunting—and perhaps somewhat disheartening—statistics on chronic illnesses, including obesity and diabetes, in the United States and around the world, research has shown that taking small steps to achieving a healthy weight and maintaining an active lifestyle can make a dramatic difference on the course of your life. According to the USDA, healthier diets such as plant-based eating could prevent about $71 billion in yearly health care costs, lost productivity, and premature deaths. This number is staggering when you consider that the change could be as small as choosing a hearty salad instead of a steak for dinner!

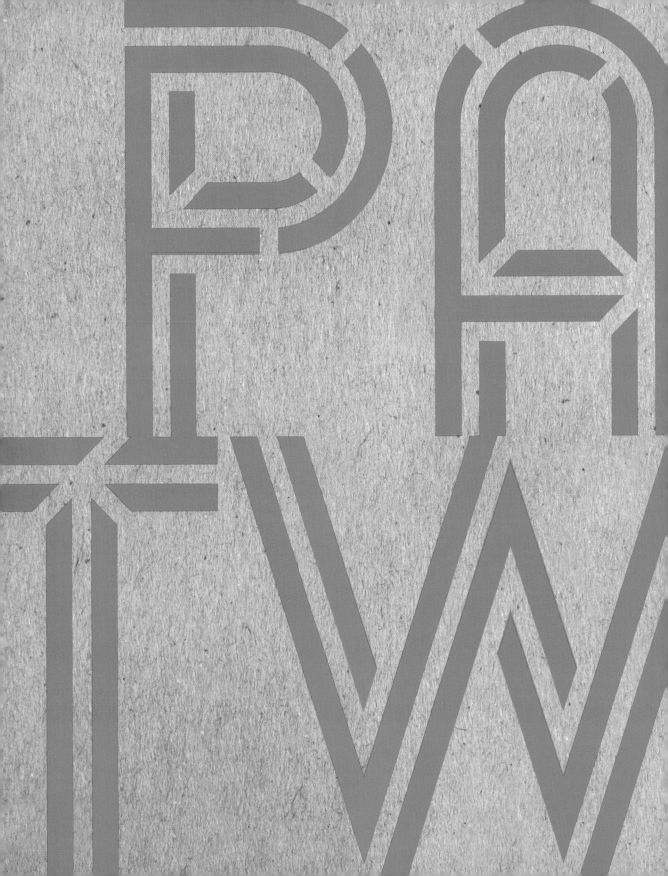

NOW IT'S TIME TO PUT THESE LAWS INTO ACTION in your life. You're going to do that in an easy, fun incremental fashion with three transitional tiers. Here is an overview about how they work. I understand that everyone is coming to the Greenprint from a different starting point. Where you begin depends on where you are right now. Many of you have never really considered going 100 percent plant-based—until now. You're ready to eat more plants, make the switch, eat less of everything else (Law #1) and start today (Law #14). But exactly *where* do you start?

What's unique about the Greenprint diet is that it helps you structure your switch to plant-based eating through the following transitional tiers, all of which are infused with the twenty-two Greenprint laws:

TIER 1: THE GRADUAL SHIFT //
The idea here is to start eating one plant-based meal a day for eleven days. This could be breakfast, lunch, or dinner. Your goal is simple—just one daily plant-based meal.

TIER 2: THE RAMP-UP //
Here is where you get a little more serious. Eat two plant-based meals daily for eleven days, while simultaneously cutting out the animal products that you'll miss the least.

TIER 3: THE FULL-ON //
This tier involves going 100 percent plant-based for life. Cut out all animal-derived ingredients and incorporate lots of vegetables, fruits, whole grains, beans, legumes, nuts, and seeds into your meals. On pages 188–195, I've laid out forty-four days of 100 percent plant-based meals as an example.

When you get to, and live, Tier 3, expect to be amazed. Let me share the story of Barbara Jean, who participated in our Holy Name study. Assigned initially to the vegetarian cohort, Barbara Jean is an excellent example of what happens to the body when you go full-on, as Tier 3 suggests.

"I did lose a little weight in the vegetarian group and felt more energetic," she explained. "But after two months, I got permission to switch to the vegan [plant-based] group."

That's when extraordinary changes kicked in.

"My energy level went through the roof," she said. "While working out, I felt like I was taking an upper, or something like it. But, of course, I wasn't. It was the plant-based diet pushing my stamina."

In those terms, Barbara Jean's switch to veganism had an impact. Before she switched to the vegan cohort, her vitals were:

> *Weight*: 136 pounds
>
> *Total cholesterol*: 181 (this was good; optimal levels are below 200)
>
> *LDL cholesterol*: 92 (this was good; optimal levels are below 100)
>
> *Hemoglobin A1C*: 5.6 (normal range is between 4 and 5.6—she was edging up a bit)

After twenty-two days, Barbara Jean was able to further improve her readings:

> *Weight*: 126 pounds
>
> *Total cholesterol*: 173
>
> *LDL cholesterol*: 87
>
> *Hemoglobin A1C*: 5.4

Now that the study is over, and Barbara has seen the rapid effect on her health, she has no desire to eat meat. In fact, she has developed a long list of favorite vegan foods, many of which beautifully substitute for animal products: beans of all kinds, vegan ground "beef," Chao cheese, plant-based burger patties, meatless meatballs, spaghetti

THE 22 GREENPRINT LAWS

LAW #1: Eat More Plants and Less of Everything Else

LAW #2: Nobody Ever Plans to Fail—People Just Fail to Plan

LAW #3: Eat More, Weigh Less

LAW #4: Water Is Life Fuel

LAW #5: Protect Your Heart

LAW #6: Take Care of Your Mind

LAW #7: Fast for Health and Longevity

LAW #8: Think About the Earth Before You Eat

LAW #9: Love Food That Loves You Back

LAW #10: Movement Begets Movement

LAW #11: Trash Must Be Taken Out

LAW #12: The World Doesn't Need Us to Survive—We Need the World to Survive

LAW #13: Change Starts with You

LAW #14: The Best Starting Point Is Today

LAW #15: Perfection Can Be the Enemy of Progress

LAW #16: Listen to Your Body

LAW #17: Focus on What You Can Eat, Not What You Can't

LAW #18: Plants Have All the Power We Need

LAW #19: A Behavior That Is Rewarded Will Be Repeated

LAW #20: You Cannot Give What You Do Not Have

LAW #21: Bring Mindfulness to Eating

LAW #22: Practice *Kaizen*

squash, zoodles, vegan sour cream, hummus instead of mayonnaise, and many more.

"I've come across lots of nutritionally beneficial and tasty vegan recipes that I'll continue to cook."

The take-home message here is that it is easier to get to, and stay on, Tier 1, once you start living it.

MAKING THE TRANSITION

In a stepwise fashion, moving from Tier 1 to Tier 3, you can gradually cut down on all animal products or remove one animal-based food group at a time. But if you want to dive right in, feel free to skip to Tier 3!

I'm here to meet you where you are. Information and programs that don't take *you* into account can't work for long, because you are what makes a program work. You are the energy behind the machine. You are the power that lights the way to your transformation. That's the beauty of living the Greenprint laws and doing the Greenprint diet: You are in charge.

Wherever you are right now, let these tiers ease your transition and transformation—and help you find a sense of peace and balance.

GETTING READY

Transitioning to a plant-based lifestyle can seem daunting and scary. I get that. I grew up in Miami, where regular meals for our Cuban family included pork, chicken, or beef. I can't even remember a meal during my childhood and teenage years that didn't include one of those animal-based foods. So yes, I know it can be undeniably overwhelming, but only if you try to do it all at once.

Remember Law #22, "Practice *kaizen*"? If you focus on making one change at a time, the progression to a plant-based lifestyle will feel quite natural. I certainly commend new plant-based eaters who go 100 percent overnight, but this is certainly not how it happens for the majority of us—not even for me.

Early in my journey, I realized that a plant-based diet was really about what I *added*, not what I took away. The more I focused on all the new foods I was trying, the less I felt like I was missing out at all. My diet used to be so limited and boring, lacking in colorful produce and inspiration. I was pleasantly surprised by the wide variety of foods I could eat on a plant-based diet. It was then that I created Law #17, "Focus on what you can eat, not what you can't." Vegan, plant-based diets are so bountiful—just think of all the fruits, vegetables, beans, grains, seeds, nuts, and spices at your fingertips. Open your eyes to all the amazing foods you haven't yet tried. These are foods you will love, and they will love you back (Law #9).

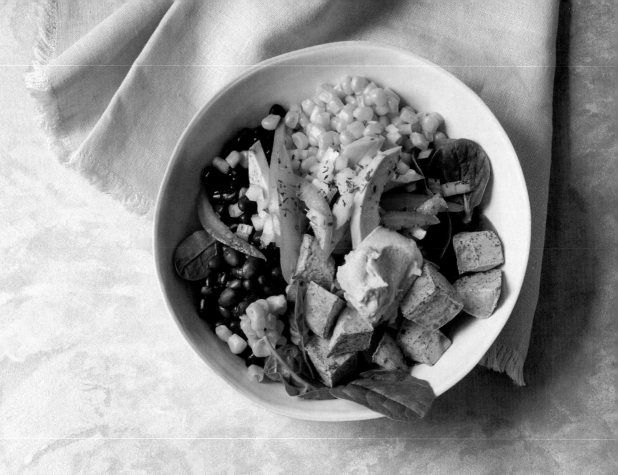

The point is that it's important to go at your own pace and to decide what approach works best for you.

Before you start, be sure to take an initial "snapshot" of your health by measuring your metrics, including your:

// Weight

// Blood pressure

// Cholesterol level

// Blood sugar (fasting)

// Energy level and endurance

// Strength

// Sex drive

// Sleep quality

Tracking these measures helps quantify the effect of the Greenprint on your life and will help you evaluate the changes you see and experience while following the program. Write down your starting numbers in a journal and periodically revisit them as you go through the three tiers. Doing so is a vital part of Law #16, "Listen to your body."

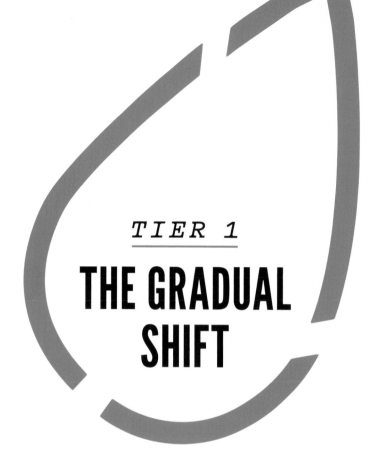

TIER 1
THE GRADUAL SHIFT

PART
TWO

—

TIER 1

—

THE GRADUAL
SHIFT

—

PAGE
170

ON TIER 1, EAT ONE PLANT-BASED MEAL DAILY FOR ELEVEN DAYS.
It could be breakfast, lunch, or dinner—or you can mix it up, eating your
plant-based meal at breakfast one day, lunch the next, and dinner the
next, and so on, for example.

Whichever meal you choose, make sure it's the one that is easiest
for you to make plant-based. You might already be enjoying a green
smoothie or cereal with nondairy milk for breakfast—stay with that.
Maybe you already pack a salad to take to work—instead of topping
it with tuna or chicken, add some chickpeas and you're all set. As for
dinner, try making one of your favorite dishes with plant-based proteins
rather than meat. A good example is chili: Substitute black beans for
ground beef, and you won't even know the difference.

Planning your daily plant meal is key. It ensures that you'll like the dish you're going to eat and look forward to eating it. Food can be healthy and plant-based, but it also needs to be appetizing. You need to enjoy it, too.

While you're on Tier 1, begin to eliminate one or two animal-based food groups. These could be:

Red meat (beef, lamb, pork, and other red meat)

Chicken and poultry

Fish and shellfish

Cheese

Eggs

Honey

Butter, cream, and other dairy products

During these eleven days, learn as much as you can about plant-based living—its benefits, how to nourish your body with this style of eating, and the practices and costs behind the production of animal products. There are loads of reasons to move toward a plant-based diet, but focus on finding your personal reasons. Revisit the laws. They offer valuable insights and support, and will help you feel more confident in your transition.

Keep your small-step *kaizen* goals in mind: one plant-based meal daily for eleven days, and the elimination of one or two animal-based food groups. That's it. What could be easier?

YOUR DAILY STRATEGY ON TIER 1:
EASY MEAL CHOICES AND RECOMMENDED RECIPES FOR TIER 1

BREAKFAST

Gluten-free whole-grain toast with nut butter, accompanied by a bowl of fresh chopped fruit

Hot cereal with nut milk, topped with a sliced banana

1 cup vegan yogurt mixed with fresh berries and topped with chopped raw almonds and sunflower seeds

Simple green smoothie: 1 cup nut milk, 1 scoop vegan protein powder, handful of spinach, and 1 cup frozen unsweetened berries

1 cup granola with nut milk and a piece of fresh fruit

Blended vegetable juice: handful of baby kale, handful of baby spinach, 1 pear (peeled and chopped), 1 celery stalk (chopped), 1/2 cucumber (peeled and chopped), and water as needed for blending

Mashed avocado on gluten-free whole-grain toast, topped with raw sunflower seeds

TIER 1 BREAKFAST RECIPES TO TRY

Almond Butter and Banana Green Smoothie (page 198)

Pumpkin Pie Smoothie (page 199)

Apple Pie Smoothie (page 200)

Banana-Walnut Overnight Oats (page 201)

LUNCH

Hummus and chopped fresh veggies

Salad bar items like chickpeas and three bean salad over lettuce

Vegan lentil soup (canned)

Vegetable burger with a green side salad and dressing

Mashed avocado and sprouts on a whole-grain pita with 1 cup vegan bean soup (canned)

Hummus sandwich on gluten-free whole-grain bread with grated carrots and thinly sliced cucumbers

Garden salad (with lots of salad veggies) topped with dressing and mixed with quinoa

TIER 1 LUNCH RECIPES TO TRY

Herbed White Bean and Pea Salad (page 202)

Raw Broccoli Salad (page 203)

Raw Veggie Salad or Raw Rainbow Salad (pages 204–205)

Vegan Minestrone Soup (page 206)

DINNER

Stir-fried Asian veggies over quinoa

Beans and rice

Vegan chili (canned)

Vegan fajitas: sautéed bell peppers, onions, and eggplant served in whole-grain tortillas and topped with salsa and jalapeños

Mashed sweet potato, black beans, and kale side salad

Vegan cauliflower pizza (store-bought) and green side salad

Pasta topped with prepared marinara sauce, steamed zucchini, and sautéed onions

TIER 1 DINNER RECIPES TO TRY

Maggie's Spicy Eggplant Stir-Fry (page 207)

Avocado and Broccoli Lettuce Cups (page 208)

Black Bean and Kale Wrap (page 211)

TIER 2

THE RAMP-UP

LET'S TAKE IT UP A NOTCH! For the next eleven days, commit to eating two plant-based meals daily. Again, these could be breakfast and lunch, or breakfast and dinner, or lunch and dinner—whatever combination works for you. Plan out which meals you'll select for plant-based eating.

In Tier 1, you cut out one or two animal-based food groups. On Tier 2, continue to slowly lessen your consumption of animal products while simultaneously increasing the number of plant-based foods in your diet. Are there animal products you won't miss in your diet? Eliminate those over the next eleven days.

Stay mindful about your motivation to change. When you know exactly *why* you want to go 100 percent plant-based, you simply won't stray from the lifestyle. This is why it is so important to learn the benefits of a plant-based lifestyle and the effects eating animal products can have on your health and the environment. Once this gets in your mind and heart, there's no turning back. The twenty-two laws will help you.

PART
TWO

—

TIER 2

—

THE
RAMP-UP

—

PAGE

173

YOUR DAILY STRATEGY ON TIER 2:

EASY MEAL CHOICES AND RECOMMENDED RECIPES FOR TIER 2

Review the meal suggestions listed for breakfast, lunch, and dinner. Double up from Tier 1: Choose two meals daily that are plant-based and enjoy those over the next eleven days.

Tier 2 is the right time to start doing more plant-based cooking. Start with the recipes in this book. They will give you inspiration and amazing meal ideas, and you'll discover just how incredibly tasty and creative plant-based meals can be! This was key to my success, and one of the first things I tell others to do, too. Identify at least three recipes from Tier 1 and Tier 2 that you'll enjoy and can prepare regularly over the next eleven days.

Also, experiment with converting some of your favorite recipes to plant-based recipes. Enjoy bean burritos using refried beans instead of beef, veggie burgers instead of hamburgers, and grilled veggies instead of grilled chicken in sandwiches. Many soups, stews, and casseroles can be turned into vegan dishes with a few simple changes.

TIER 2 BREAKFAST
RECIPES TO TRY

Peanut Butter Smoothie Bowl (page 212)

Homemade Granola (page 213)

Chia Oat Peanut Butter Parfait (page 215)

Blueberry Bliss Bowl (page 216)

Avocado Toast with Sunflower Seeds and Sprouts (page 218)

TIER 2 LUNCH
RECIPES TO TRY

Hearts of Palm and Sweet Pea Pasta Salad (page 217)

Shredded Brussels Sprouts Salad (page 220)

Sweet Potato Toast with Hummus and Broccoli Sprouts (page 221)

Mexican-Inspired Bean Salad (page 223)

Split Pea Soup (page 224)

Chickpea No-Tuna Salad Sandwich (page 232)

Chickpea and Avocado Burgers (page 235)

PART
TWO

TIER 2

THE
RAMP-UP

PAGE
174

TIER 2 DINNER
RECIPES TO TRY

Chickpea and Avocado Burgers (page 235)

Spinach and Mushroom Gnocchi with Walnut
Meat (page 227)

Loaded Sweet Potato (page 228)

Mushroom "Chorizo" Lettuce Tacos
(page 231)

Once you've completed Tiers 1 and 2, you've
got a lot of plant-eating under your belt.
Along the way, you've begun to form new
habits and reset your body and mind. When
I was studying psychology in college, I
discovered that many psychologists believe
it takes around twenty-one days to make or
break a habit. The more often you engage
in a specific behavior, the more pathways
your brain builds to support that behavior.
Scientists call this "neuroplasticity": the
ability of your brain to alter its connections
and responses to new information and
actions that it receives.

So you are well under way to changing
your lifestyle for good and becoming the
best version of you. Next you've got to take it
further: forty-four days of 100 percent plant-
based eating. That's what Tier 3 is all about,
and you're ready for it!

PART
TWO

—

TIER 2

—

THE
RAMP-UP

—

PAGE
175

TRANSITIONAL TIPS

When transitioning to a 100 percent plant-based diet, one of the first—and easiest—changes people make is to cut out dairy and eggs. As one of my clients who made the switch told me, "No more nasal allergies, no more sinus infections, and my acne has completely disappeared. Had I known about these side benefits, I would've gone a hundred percent plant-based years ago!"

THERE ARE SO MANY HEALTHY VEGAN SWAPS, YOU WILL **ABSOLUTELY NOT MISS** *DAIRY AND EGGS.*

REPLACING EGGS

How you choose to replace eggs depends on what they're being used in (and used for). Mashed ripe banana or applesauce can both easily be used in recipes in place of eggs; $1/4$ cup nondairy yogurt is another good substitute. However, if the egg is needed to "bind" ingredients, you'll need to up your game:

FLAX EGGS: For each egg in the recipe, mix 1 tablespoon ground flaxseed with 3 tablespoons warm water. Let sit for a few minutes before using in the recipe.

CHIA EGGS: For each egg in the recipe, mix 1 tablespoon chia seeds with $2 1/2$ tablespoons warm water. Let sit for a few minutes, until the mixture becomes a bit "gummy," before using in the recipe. (You can also grind the chia seeds first to reduce their appearance in your baked goodies.)

These egg replacers are great for recipes like cookies and even puddings. However, if the egg in your original recipe is used for leavening (meaning it helps your final product to rise, as in muffins or quick breads), then you need something a bit lighter:

2 teaspoons baking soda
+ 2 tablespoons warm water

1 teaspoon baking powder
+ 1 teaspoon apple cider vinegar.

Flax eggs as described above.

REPLACING BUTTER AND OIL

There are more vegan butters than ever before. From coconut butter and whipped spreads to my current favorite, Miyoko's Vegan Butter, you will never miss the smell of melted butter on your hot breakfast toast.

For optimal homemade alternatives, even if an ingredient is already vegan (such as vegetable oil), you can still make your recipe healthier! Here are a few common substitutes for butter (or margarine) and oil:

BUTTER REPLACERS: equal quantity of nondairy spread, coconut oil, olive oil, vegan shortening, avocado puree; 3/4 cup prunes blended with 1/4 cup water per 1 cup (2 sticks) butter

ONE-ON-ONE OIL REPLACERS: mashed banana, 2 to 3 teaspoons chia seeds, or melted coconut oil mixed with 1 cup water

Be aware of the flavor of what you are using as a replacer. For example, avocado puree might work well for a dark, savory bread, but not so well in a light-colored cake.

SWEETENERS

Whether a recipe calls for honey, sugar, brown sugar, or another sweetener, you can choose to up its nutrient value by swapping out the sweetener for something healthier, less calorie-dense, and with a lower glycemic index. Common substitutions include:

1/2 teaspoon pure vanilla extract for 2 tablespoons of sugar

Applesauce for sugar (equal quantities)

Agave nectar or maple syrup for honey (equal quantities)

Coconut sugar for sugar (equal quantities)

You could also try adding cinnamon and reducing the overall quantity of sugar or sweetener in a recipe, because recipes are often much sweeter than necessary to begin with.

MILK AND CREAM

I'm always amazed when I see the mammoth wall of nondairy milk in my grocery store. It's taking over! Use nondairy milks, such as almond milk, rice milk, coconut milk, cashew milk, or hemp seed milk, to name just a few, in place of cow's milk in your smoothies, over cereal, and for other basic needs. It's pretty easy to simply sub in nondairy milk when regular milk is called for, but what about other forms of milk, or more complex recipes? Here are a few other substitutions you can employ:

BUTTERMILK: Whisk together 1 cup nondairy milk and 2 teaspoons cider vinegar or fresh lemon juice and let sit for 10 minutes. Or mix equal parts vegan sour cream and water.

EVAPORATED MILK: Chill a can of full-fat coconut milk overnight. Scoop out the thick white cream and use it in place of evaporated milk.

WHIPPED CREAM: Chill a can of full-fat coconut milk overnight. Scoop the thick white cream into a bowl and whisk until it holds soft peaks.

CHEESE: Make cashew cheese, or purchase it at specialty grocery stores that cater to vegans. It can be substituted for dairy cheese in most recipes.

YOGURT: Try vegan yogurt if you're a yogurt lover.

THE FULL-ON

FOR THE NEXT FORTY-FOUR DAYS, eat three plant-based meals and snacks every day—in other words, you'll go 100 percent plant-based. I'll give you sample menus to help you during your transition.

Now's the time to remove any remaining animal-based foods from your diet. Focus on adding more plant-based protein sources instead. Pay attention to ingredient lists and avoid foods containing gelatin, rennet, and other animal products like dairy and eggs.

As part of your new adventure, visit vegan-friendly restaurants. See the Resources section (page 297) for suggestions. Try ethnic restaurants, which tend to have many plant-based choices. Here are just a few examples: Chinese—veggie stir-fry, garlic eggplant, or fried tofu; Thai—veggie pad thai, coconut curry; Japanese—veggie sushi, edamame, miso soup (be careful because some Asian foods contain fish sauce); Ethiopian—lentils, collard greens, yellow split beans; Indian—chana masala, aloo gobi, dal, veggie samosas; Mediterranean—hummus, stuffed grape leaves, baba ghanoush; Mexican—bean burritos or tacos (just make sure they are not cooked in lard).

PART
TWO

—

TIER 3

—

THE
FULL-ON

—

PAGE
178

YOUR DAILY STRATEGY ON TIER 3:
EASY MEAL CHOICES AND RECOMMENDED RECIPES FOR TIER 3

As you continue on your plant-based journey, I've got some meal-planning tools to help you map out your success. People new to plant-based eating want to know how much to eat in order to achieve a leaner, healthier body and how to create meals that accomplish that goal.

THE GREENPRINT PORTIONS

First, how much of each group of plant foods should you eat daily? Generally, the daily breakdown looks like this:

Grains: up to 1 1/2 cups cooked

Beans and legumes: up to 2 cups cooked

Starchy vegetables (such as potatoes or sweet potatoes): 1/2 cup to 1 cup, or 1 whole starchy vegetable

Greens and other vegetables: unlimited quantities; try to eat 1 to 2 cups of leafy green vegetables

Nuts, nut butters, seeds, and seed butters: 1 to 2 tablespoons

Fruit: 1 to 3 servings (1 piece of fresh fruit, 1 cup berries or chopped fresh fruit)

Healthy fats and oils: 1 tablespoon oil, 1/4 to 1/2 avocado, or 10 olives

THE GREENPRINT PLATE

Put all this together by visualizing your Greenprint plate at meals. It should look something like this:

Half your plate (50 percent) should be filled with vegetables. Think: broccoli, cauliflower, asparagus, green beans, tomatoes, as well as leafy green veggies like spinach and kale. Salads are included here.

One-quarter of your plate (25 percent) should be plant proteins: beans and legumes, or a combination of these with nuts and seeds.

15 percent can be cooked grains or starchy veggies.

The rest of the plate is devoted to healthy fats.

Your plate may not look like this at every meal, but it's a good guideline for building a healthy plant-based meal.

THE GREENPRINT PANTRY

Be a 100 percent plant-based shopper. Go to the store and buy all the plant-based foods you can get your hands on! Here's what to stock up on:

PRODUCE

VEGETABLES
(fresh and frozen)

Leafy green vegetables (kale, spinach, arugula, lettuces, and so forth)

Other veggies (broccoli, cauliflower, Brussels sprouts, onions, tomatoes, celery, bell peppers, summer squash, green beans, carrots, etc.)

STARCHY VEGETABLES
(fresh and frozen)

Beets

Corn

Parsnips

Peas

Potatoes

Pumpkin

Sweet potatoes

Winter squash

FRUIT

Avocados

Bananas and other tropical fruits

Berries

Citrus fruits

Melons

Stone fruits (peach, plums, nectarines)

GRAINS

Healthy whole grains make a great base or side dish and provide protein and carbohydrates. For breakfast, lunch, or dinner, keep the following items on hand:

Amaranth

Brown rice

Buckwheat

Millet

Oats

Quinoa

FLOURS

Almond flour

Chickpea flour

Gluten-free flour blend

BEANS AND LEGUMES

Dried or canned beans and legumes can provide a base for most meals: chili, masala, soups, curries, sauces, and other great dishes. Look for cans without BPA linings or opt for glass jars. (BPA is a toxin that interrupts hormonal function in the body.)

Black beans

Cannellini beans

Chickpeas (garbanzo beans)

Kidney beans

Lentils

Navy beans

Pinto beans

Split peas

PART
TWO

—

TIER 3

—

THE
FULL-ON

PAGE
180

WATCH OUT

FOR SOME PLANT FOODS

Not all plant-based whole foods are created equal—which is why it's important to know how to swap out foods with a less complete nutritional profile for more nutrient-dense options. Doing so will help you get more nutrients, feel more full, and reduce cravings. Here are a few healthy plant swaps you can try out:

WHITE POTATOES

Instead of white potatoes (which are still healthy in moderation), eat more sweet potatoes instead—you'll get more fiber (three times as much), as well as a ton of vitamin A. Enjoy oven-baked sweet potatoes fries or add diced sweet potatoes to your favorite soups or quinoa dishes.

CROUTONS

Addicted to the crunch that croutons add to your salads? Try swapping out your traditional high-cholesterol croutons for fresh or roasted nuts (try almonds, cashews, or pecans).

WHITE RICE

Sense a theme? White foods, in general, have less nutritional value than more colorful alternatives. Try replacing white rice with quinoa—a whole protein with higher fiber and fewer carbohydrates. (Quinoa is a great alternative for standard wheat flour–based pasta, as well.) And if you're looking for a low-carb option, try riced cauliflower, which is available in the frozen foods section of your grocery store.

CEREAL

Most cereals are loaded with sugar and empty carbohydrates. A warm bowl of oatmeal, with a few nuts and fruit thrown on top, can offer you a healthier breakfast with a well-rounded nutritional profile.

ORANGE JUICE

Nothing beats fresh juice, but by discarding the flesh, you're also throwing away a lot of nutrients. Having a whole-fruit smoothie instead will give you longer-term satisfaction and provide your body with the fuel it needs to get through the day. You can maximize your smoothie's benefits by including healthy add-ins like chia seeds, almond butter, or a handful of greens. Blending a scoop of vegan protein powder into your smoothie gives you an added boost to start your day off strong.

FAUX MEAT

Before they become "meat," soy-based products undergo heavy processing and often use GMO products. You can easily make delicious, high-protein meat alternatives using wild rice, nuts, beans, lentils, quinoa, and sweet potato.

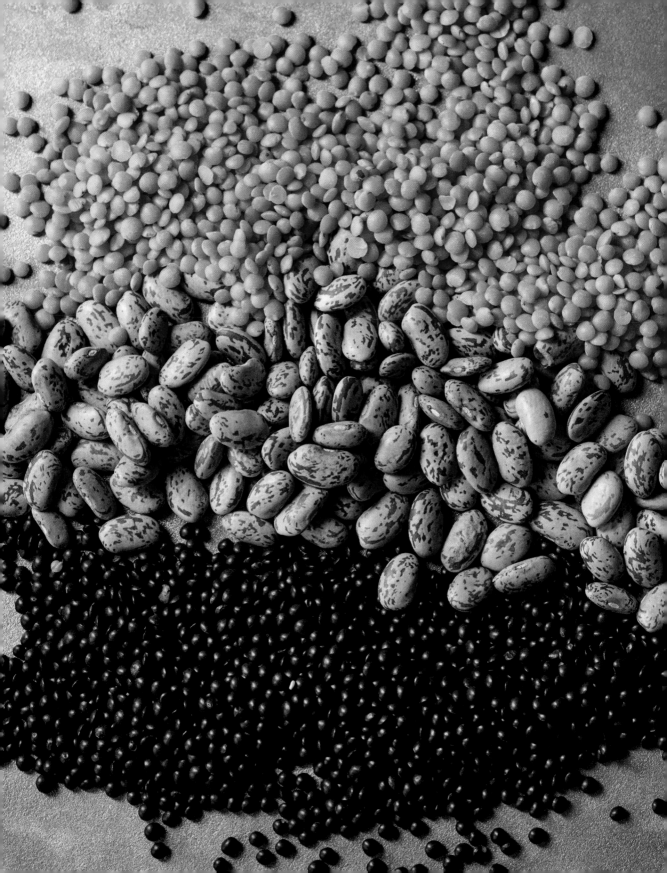

NUTS AND SEEDS

Including seeds and nuts in your meals adds protein and trace minerals, among other nutrients. Nuts and seeds don't stay fresh forever; depending on the nut or seed, they last anywhere between six months and two years. It's a good idea to check expiration dates and cycle out your stock regularly, so they don't get stale or rancid. Or put them in the fridge once you've opened a new container.

Some suggestions include:

Almonds

Cashews

Chia seeds

Flaxseeds

Hemp seeds

Nut butters

Peanuts (technically a legume)

Pecans

Pine nuts

Pumpkin seeds

Sesame seeds

Sunflower seeds

Vegan trail mix

Walnuts

NUT MILKS

Almond milk

Almond-coconut milk blend

Cashew milk

Coconut milk

DRIED FRUITS AND VEGETABLES

Apples (dried)

Apricots (dried)

Cranberries

Currants

Dates

Figs

Prunes

Raisins

Shiitakes and other mushrooms

Sun-dried tomatoes

HERBS AND SPICES

Besides adding flavor to your meal, spices and herbs contain essential micronutrients. Although fresh herbs are best, keep a stock of dried herbs on hand and use them to increase the flavor of pretty much any meal so you can enjoy your vegan dishes, rather than suffering through them. For sweet dishes, try cinnamon, ginger, vanilla, or even a dash of cayenne pepper. Other suggestions include the standby thyme, oregano, basil, paprika, and cumin.

Basil, dried

Black peppercorns, for grinding

Cayenne pepper

Chili powder

Cinnamon, ground

Coriander, ground and whole seeds

Cumin, ground and whole seeds

Curry powder

Dulse flakes

Garlic powder

Nutmeg, whole seeds for grating fresh

Onion powder

Oregano, dried

Paprika, regular

Paprika, smoked

Parsley flakes, dried

Pumpkin pie spice

Sea salt

Thyme, dried

Turmeric, ground

Vanilla extract, pure

HEALTHY FATS

Avocados

Coconut oil

Grapeseed oil

Olive oil

Olives

Sesame oil

Vegan salad dressings

VINEGAR

Balsamic vinegar

Cider vinegar

Distilled white vinegar

Red wine vinegar

Rice vinegar

CONDIMENTS/ MISCELLANEOUS

Agave nectar

Applesauce, unsweetened

Baking powder, gluten-free

Baking soda

Barbecue sauce

Coconut aminos

Coconut amino–based teriyaki sauce

Coconut wraps

Cornstarch

Hot sauce or sriracha

Liquid smoke

Maple syrup, pure

Mayonnaise, vegan

Mustard, Dijon

Mustard, stone-ground

Nutritional yeast

Tahini

Tomato paste

Vanilla protein powder, vegan

Vegetable broth

Many of these items may already be in your pantry, so it's just a matter of rounding out what you have with a few additional ingredients. While you are surveying your pantry, be sure to clear out any items you won't need once you switch to a plant-based diet. Look out for things that are heavily processed and those that contain animal products. Once you have your pantry in order, you'll be all set for a long and healthy plant-based life.

VEGAN BOWLS

Are you having a hard time putting together healthy lunches? Stuck for a simple, nutritious dinner? Then vegan bowls might be just what you've been missing. They're easy to make and delicious to eat—all you have to do is pick a few ingredients and put them together. Here's how:

STEP 1

CHOOSE
VEGGIES

They can be fresh, steamed, grilled, or roasted, but you'll want lots of veggies for your vegan bowls. Aim for a range of colors in each bowl—and don't forget your leafy greens! Any veggies will do, even if it's just leftovers from the night before or frozen vegetables.

STEP 2

CHOOSE
CARBS

Steer yourself toward complex carbs and away from simple carbs (such as white rice, plain pasta, white potatoes, etc.). Some good options include quinoa, wild rice, and sweet potatoes. This is also a great time to try some other grains like millet or sorghum. Keep your serving of grains to about 1/2 cup.

STEP 3

ADD
PROTEIN

Your veggies and complex carbs already contain some protein, but you can boost the protein content with the addition of beans, legumes, nuts, and/or seeds. Delicious options include lentils, chickpeas, sliced almonds, hemp seeds, and pumpkin seeds. Stick to servings of about 1/2 cup for beans and legumes and 1/4 cup for nuts and seeds.

STEP 4

GO FOR
HEALTHY FATS

Fats are an important part of any diet and can help to fill out your vegan bowl. Some ideas include olive oil, tahini, and avocado. If you have already added fats (such as hemp hearts, nuts, or seeds), be aware of how much additional fat you add to your bowl.

STEP 5

FLAVOR!

Add some flavor to your bowl with herbs, spices, or dressings. Think: fresh lemon juice, chopped fresh cilantro, a sprinkle of curry powder, or a dressing.

THE 44-DAY FULL-ON GREENPRINT DIET

The following plan is a simple and adaptable guide to making the full transition to 100 percent plant-based eating. It covers forty-four days of meals. To be successful:

// Try to eat as closely to the meal plan as possible. It's fine to substitute foods as long as they are 100 percent whole plant foods. Avoid processed vegan foods.

// Plan and build your meals according to the portion and plate guidelines described on page 179.

// Don't drink any alcoholic beverages, for three reasons:

1 You'll be drinking empty calories.

2 Alcohol leads to dehydration, which makes you hungrier and can lower your willpower, leading to bad food choices.

3 You will start to fall into old habits and crave foods you've eliminated from your diet. Later on, after you've experienced the benefits of plant-based eating, feel free to enjoy the occasional glass of beer, wine, or liquor as part of your new healthy lifestyle.

// Be sure to keep yourself well hydrated by drinking plenty of water throughout the day. Other permissible beverages are tea, herbal tea, coffee, and unsweetened coconut water.

// Follow my recommendations for intermittent fasting by going 14 to 16 hours without food overnight.

// Eat up to 80 percent fullness at every meal; do not overload or otherwise stuff your stomach.

GET STARTED!

BREAKFAST EVERY DAY

// A plant-based smoothie (see pages 198–200)

// A whole-grain cereal such as quinoa, oatmeal, or granola with nut milk and a serving of fresh fruit

// Mashed avocado on gluten-free whole-grain toast with a serving of fresh fruit

// Plant-based breakfast bowl

// Any favorite plant-based breakfast

TIER 3 BREAKFAST RECIPES:

Banana-Nut Quinoa Bowl (page 236)

Almond Granola Oat Cup (page 238)

Dried Fruit Brown Rice Porridge (page 240)

Kale Breakfast Salad (page 243)

Spinach Tortilla (Spinach Omelet) (page 245)

Almond Butter and Blueberry Sweet Potato Toast (page 246)

BLT Breakfast Sandwich (page 249)

PART
TWO

———

TIER 3

———

THE
FULL-ON

———

PAGE
186

PART
TWO

—

TIER 3

—

THE
FULL-ON

—

PAGE

187

DAY 1

LUNCH // Spiralized zucchini mixed with quinoa and your choice of salad dressing

AFTERNOON SNACK // Fresh fruit with a dollop of nut butter

DINNER // *Build-your-own burrito:* Whole-grain wraps, pinto or black beans, some salsa, and a handful of at least two veggies such as chopped onion, chopped bell peppers, sliced jalapeños, and/or shredded lettuce

DAY 2

LUNCH // Arugula with sliced almonds, grapes, and chopped broccoli, drizzled with vinaigrette

AFTERNOON SNACK // Handful of roasted chickpeas

DINNER // Black beans, kale, and quinoa, topped with salsa and avocado slices

DAY 3

LUNCH // Black bean burger on a gluten-free whole-grain bun with fresh spinach and sun-dried tomatoes

AFTERNOON SNACK // A vegan nut-and-fruit bar

DINNER // Vegan chili over cooked quinoa

DAY 4

LUNCH // Leftover black bean burger from day 3

AFTERNOON SNACK // Bowl of edamame

DINNER // *Chickpea stir-fry:* chickpeas, bell peppers, chopped onions, and shredded cabbage, cooked with coconut aminos and served over rice or quinoa

DAY 5

LUNCH // Leftover chickpea stir-fry from day 4

AFTERNOON SNACK // Toasted gluten-free pita with salsa and guacamole

DINNER // Veggie sushi rolls, miso soup, and edamame

DAY 6

LUNCH // Baked sweet potato topped with pinto beans, bell peppers, spinach, and pineapple salsa

AFTERNOON SNACK // ¼ cup hummus with fresh vegetables for dipping (carrots, celery, romaine leaves, bell pepper, etc.)

DINNER // Black bean chili with green side salad, drizzled with salad dressing

DAY 7

LUNCH // ¼ cup black bean hummus with celery, carrots, and cucumbers for dipping, a handful of almonds, and 1 cup grapes

AFTERNOON SNACK // A piece of fresh fruit

DINNER // Leftover black bean chili from day 6 with green side salad, drizzled with salad dressing

DAY 8

LUNCH // Beans and rice

AFTERNOON SNACK //
¼ cup black bean hummus with fresh vegetables for dipping (carrots, celery, romaine leaves, bell pepper, etc.)

DINNER // *Chickpea pasta with pesto:* Sautéed zucchini, eggplant, onions, and mushrooms, mixed with chickpea pasta and tossed with pesto sauce

DAY 9

LUNCH // Leftover chickpea pasta with pesto from day 8

AFTERNOON SNACK //
¼ cup black bean hummus with fresh vegetables for dipping (carrots, celery, romaine leaves, bell pepper, etc.)

DINNER // Baked sweet potato with 1 tablespoon melted coconut oil, ½ cup black beans, and steamed greens as desired (or a green side salad)

DAY 10

LUNCH // *Large salad:* at least 3 cups greens with salad veggies such as onions and tomatoes, 3 tablespoons pumpkin or hemp seeds, and dressing of your choice

AFTERNOON SNACK //
1 ounce almonds and 3 tablespoons raisins

DINNER // Quinoa with cooked broccoli and cauliflower, topped with sriracha

DAY 11

LUNCH // *Large salad:* at least 3 cups greens (whichever you like), ½ cup beans or lentils, 2 tablespoons sliced almonds, vegetables, and dressing of your choice

AFTERNOON SNACK //
Apple with 2 tablespoons almond butter

DINNER // Vegan cauliflower pizza (store-bought) with green side salad, drizzled with salad dressing

DAY 12

LUNCH // *Sandwich wrap:* mashed avocado on a gluten-free pita or tortilla, filled with sprouts, spinach, sliced cherry tomatoes, or other veggies

AFTERNOON SNACK //
1 cup almond milk blended with 1 scoop vegan vanilla protein powder and a few ice cubes

DINNER // *Vegan fajitas:* sautéed bell peppers, onions, and eggplant served in whole-grain tortillas and topped with salsa and jalapeños

DAY 13

LUNCH // Leftover vegan fajitas from day 12

AFTERNOON SNACK //
¼ cup vegan trail mix, or 2 tablespoons raw almonds or cashews and 2 tablespoons dried fruit

DINNER // 1 cup cooked quinoa, brown rice, or millet, served with ½ cup chopped avocado, 1 cup steamed greens, and dressing of your choice

DAY 14

LUNCH // Large lettuce or collard leaves filled with beans, chopped veggies, and salsa or guacamole

AFTERNOON SNACK // Handful of roasted chickpeas

DINNER // Spiralized zucchini and yellow squash, topped with diced tomatoes, 1 (15-ounce) can black beans (drained and rinsed), and some avocado slices

DAY 15

LUNCH // Leftover lettuce wraps

AFTERNOON SNACK // 1 piece of fresh fruit

DINNER // Leftover spiralized zucchini and yellow squash from day 14

DAY 16

LUNCH // *Sandwich wrap:* Mashed avocado on a gluten-free pita or tortilla, filled with sprouts, spinach, sliced cherry tomatoes, or other veggies

AFTERNOON SNACK // ¼ cup hummus with fresh vegetables for dipping (carrots, celery, romaine leaves, bell pepper, etc.)

DINNER // *Beans, greens, and grains:* sautéed greens mixed with cooked beans and grains, topped with hot sauce

DAY 17

LUNCH // Beans and rice

AFTERNOON SNACK // ¼ cup raw trail mix

DINNER // Leftover beans, greens, and grains from day 16

DAY 18

LUNCH // Leftover beans and rice from day 17

AFTERNOON SNACK // 3 tablespoons peanut butter with celery sticks

DINNER // *Vegan fajitas:* sautéed bell peppers, onions, and eggplant served in whole-grain tortillas and topped with salsa and jalapeños

DAY 19

LUNCH // Large lettuce or collard leaves filled with beans, chopped veggies, and salsa or guacamole

AFTERNOON SNACK // 1 piece of fresh fruit

DINNER // Lentil soup (canned) with a side of steamed greens and sliced fresh tomato

LUNCHBOXES

You might be wondering what kinds of healthy
plant-based meals you can pack for lunch.
Don't worry—I have some ideas.

SANDWICHES AND ROLLS

Get creative with filling ingredients, as well as
what you use on the outside—gluten-free vegan
bread, tortillas, crackers, lettuce leaves, collard
greens, etc. Here are some combinations to
consider:

Avocado and tomato

Sunflower seed butter and banana

Hummus and cucumber

Spinach and vegan cheese quesadilla

Veggie wrap

Walnut tacos

Veggie burger

RICE BOWLS AND SALADS

Rice bowls, noodle bowls, and salads all make
for great packed lunches. Plus, you can get
inventive with ingredients and sauces, or just
use whatever you have on hand, such as:

Quinoa, millet

Red rice, wild rice, brown rice

Shredded lettuce, kale, cabbage, carrots

Zucchini, cucumber, carrot noodles (invest in a
good spiralizer—it will save hours!)

Good toppings: crushed nuts, seeds, croutons,
dried fruit, etc.

Pasta (macaroni, fusilli, orzo, shells)

While you might not have a problem being
creative when it comes to finding great lunches,
it may be difficult to find the time to construct
lunches from scratch each day. Check out these
time-saving tips:

BIG BATCHES

Making muffins? Make a dozen or two extra and
store them in the freezer. The same goes for
quick breads and other home-baked goods.

WEEKEND WARRIOR

Do double-duty by making something on the
weekend that can also sub in for lunches during
the week. Stews and soups are perfect warming
lunches that you can make ahead of time.

LEFTOVERS!

If there's a dinner meal or two you love, why not
have it for lunch the next day as well? Pasta is a
great example.

DAY 20

LUNCH // Arugula with sliced almonds, grapes, and chopped broccoli, drizzled with vinaigrette

AFTERNOON SNACK // Fresh fruit with a dollop of nut butter

DINNER // Black beans with brown rice, served with a fresh salad drizzled with the dressing of your choice, or steamed vegetables

DAY 21

LUNCH // Leftover black beans with brown rice from day 20

AFTERNOON SNACK // Handful of roasted chickpeas

DINNER // *Build-your-own burrito:* whole-grain wraps, pinto or black beans, some salsa, and a handful of at least two veggies, such as chopped onion, chopped bell peppers, sliced jalapeños, and/or shredded lettuce

DAY 22

LUNCH // Black bean burger on gluten-free whole-grain bun with fresh spinach and sun-dried tomatoes

AFTERNOON SNACK // 1 piece of fresh fruit

DINNER // Leftover burrito from day 21

DAY 23

LUNCH // Leftover black bean burger from day 22

AFTERNOON SNACK // Handful of roasted chickpeas

DINNER // Stir-fried Asian veggies over quinoa

DAY 24

LUNCH // Leftover Asian stir-fry

AFTERNOON SNACK // 1 cup almond milk blended with 1 scoop vegan vanilla protein powder

DINNER // Grilled portobello mushrooms drizzled with balsamic vinegar, served with red kidney beans and a green side salad drizzled with salad dressing

DAY 25

LUNCH // Boiled artichoke with salad dressing for dipping and a side of quinoa

AFTERNOON SNACK // ¼ cup raw trail mix

DINNER // Vegan stuffed grape leaves (store-bought) topped with hummus, served with a small Greek salad (lettuce, sliced cucumbers, onions, kalamata olives, and Greek dressing)

DAY 26

LUNCH // Leftover boiled artichoke from day 25 with salad dressing for dipping and a side of quinoa

AFTERNOON SNACK // 2 tablespoons peanut or almond butter spread on celery sticks and topped with raisins ("ants on a log" style)

DINNER // Leftover vegan stuffed grape leaves with hummus from day 25

DAY 27

LUNCH // *Sandwich wrap:* mashed avocado on a gluten-free pita or tortilla, filled with sprouts, spinach, sliced cherry tomatoes, or other veggies

AFTERNOON SNACK // 1 piece of fresh fruit

DINNER // *Dinner salad:* raw greens and vegetables, 1 cup cooked diced sweet potatoes, 1/2 avocado (cubed), 1/2 cup cooked lentils, and dressing of your choice

DAY 28

LUNCH // *Large salad:* at least 3 cups greens (whichever you like), 1/2 cup beans or lentils, 2 tablespoons sliced almonds, vegetables, and dressing of your choice

AFTERNOON SNACK // Handful of wasabi peas

DINNER // *Spaghetti squash with cannellini:* cannellini beans, mushrooms, greens, and garlic sautéed in olive oil and tossed with cooked spaghetti squash

DAY 29

LUNCH // Leftover spaghetti squash with cannellini from day 28

AFTERNOON SNACK // Vegan yogurt and granola

DINNER // Roasted beets, sautéed greens, and brown rice topped with slivered almonds

DAY 30

LUNCH // Leftover roasted beets, greens, and brown rice from day 29

AFTERNOON SNACK // Vegan nut-and-fruit bar

DINNER // Black beans, brown rice, and sautéed poblano peppers, seasoned with hot sauce

DAY 31

LUNCH // Leftover black bean, brown rice, and poblanos from day 30

AFTERNOON SNACK // Fresh fruit with a dollop of nut butter

DINNER // Sautéed black beans, kale, and quinoa topped with salsa and sliced avocado

DAY 32

LUNCH // Large lettuce leaves or collard greens filled with beans, chopped veggies, and salsa or guacamole

AFTERNOON SNACK // 1 piece of fresh fruit

DINNER // Lentil soup (canned) with a side of steamed greens and quinoa

DAY 33

LUNCH // Black bean hummus with fresh vegetables for dipping (carrots, celery, romaine leaves, bell pepper, etc.)

AFTERNOON SNACK // 1 cup almond milk blended with 1 scoop vegan vanilla protein powder

DINNER // *Chickpea pasta with pesto:* Sautéed zucchini, eggplant, onions, and mushrooms, mixed with chickpea pasta and tossed with pesto sauce

DAY 34

LUNCH // Tomato soup with a green side salad mixed with quinoa

AFTERNOON SNACK // ¼ cup black bean hummus with fresh vegetables for dipping (carrots, celery, romaine leaves, bell pepper, etc.)

DINNER // *Vegan fajitas:* Sautéed bell peppers, onions, and eggplant in whole-grain tortillas topped with salsa and jalapeños

DAY 35

LUNCH // Leftover vegan fajitas from day 34

AFTERNOON SNACK // 2 tablespoons peanut or almond butter spread on celery sticks and topped with raisins ("ants on a log" style)

DINNER // Stir-fried Asian veggies over quinoa

DAY 36

LUNCH // Leftover stir-fry from day 35

AFTERNOON SNACK // A piece of fresh fruit

DINNER // Vegan chili (canned)

DAY 37

LUNCH // Mashed sweet potato, black beans, and kale side salad

AFTERNOON SNACK // ¼ cup raw trail mix

DINNER // Vegan cauliflower pizza (store-bought) with green side salad

DAY 38

LUNCH // *Large salad:* at least 3 cups greens (whichever you like) with ½ cup of beans or lentils, 2 tablespoons sliced almonds, vegetables, and dressing of your choice

AFTERNOON SNACK // ¼ cup raw trail mix

DINNER // Pasta topped with prepared marinara sauce, steamed zucchini, and sautéed onions

DAY 39

LUNCH // Leftover pasta from day 38

AFTERNOON SNACK // Vegan yogurt and granola

DINNER // Beans and rice with a green side salad drizzled with salad dressing

DAY 40

LUNCH // *Three bean salad:* equal amounts kidney beans, green beans, and navy beans tossed with vinaigrette, served with a side of brown rice or quinoa

AFTERNOON SNACK // Handful of wasabi peas

DINNER // Vegan stuffed grape leaves (store-bought) topped with hummus, served with a small Greek salad (lettuce, sliced cucumbers, onions, kalamata olives, and Greek dressing)

DAY 41

LUNCH // Leftover stuffed grape leaves with hummus from day 40

AFTERNOON SNACK // Handful of wasabi peas

DINNER // Black bean burger on gluten-free whole-grain bun with fresh spinach and sun-dried tomatoes

DAY 42

LUNCH // Leftover three-bean salad from day 40

AFTERNOON SNACK // 1 cup almond milk blended with 1 scoop vegan vanilla protein powder

DINNER // Spiralized zucchini and yellow squash topped with diced tomatoes, 1 (15-ounce) can black beans (drained and rinsed), and some avocado slices

DAY 43

LUNCH // *Large salad:* at least 3 cups greens (whichever you like), 3 tablespoons pumpkin or hemp seeds, and dressing of your choice

AFTERNOON SNACK // Apple with 2 tablespoons almond butter

DINNER // Leftover spiralized zucchini dish from day 42

DAY 44

LUNCH // Tomato or vegan vegetable soup (canned) with a green side salad drizzled with salad dressing

AFTERNOON SNACK // Vegan nut-and-fruit bar

DINNER // *Beans, greens, and grains:* black-eyed peas, collard greens, and barley, topped with hot sauce

THE
GREENPRINT
RECIPES

TO HELP YOU ON YOUR PLANT-BASED JOURNEY, I've created the following delicious whole-food vegan recipes. They're sorted into Tier 1, Tier 2, and Tier 3 recipes for ease of use. Tier 1 recipes are the simplest to prepare and take the least amount of prep time. Tier 2 and 3 recipes are slightly more involved, but not much.

I encourage you to try as many as you can to experience the amazing flavors of plant-based dishes. Most of the recipes make multiple servings so that you'll always have leftovers on hand the next day. As a bonus, I've included several of my favorite plant-based treat and dessert recipes. If you love sweets, you'll love these. Indulge in them a couple of times a week, if you wish. Enjoy!

PREP: **5 MINUTES** / *COOK:* **0 MINUTES** / *TOTAL:* **5 MINUTES**

ALMOND BUTTER AND BANANA GREEN SMOOTHIE

SERVES
1

Breakfast smoothies are some of my favorite ways to prepare quick nutrient-dense meals without a fuss. This smoothie is loaded with everything you need for a super start to your day, along with rich flavor that will leave you craving seconds.

// In a blender, combine the nondairy milk, banana, almond butter, and spinach and blend until smooth.

// Serve the smoothie in a mason jar, topped with the blueberries.

1 cup homemade oat milk (page 239) or store-bought almond milk

1 frozen banana

2 tablespoons crunchy almond butter

2 cups fresh spinach

¼ cup frozen blueberries, for topping

TIP

For a nut-free option, use oat milk and replace the almond butter with sunflower seed butter.

PART
TWO

—

TIER 1
RECIPES

—

PAGE
198

PUMPKIN PIE SMOOTHIE

SERVES
2

Yum! Now you can enjoy the delectable taste of pumpkin pie year-round. This recipe is filling and full of goodness, from the spices to the healthy pumpkin, plus delicious vegan protein powder to really hit the spot.

// In a blender, combine all the ingredients and blend until smooth.

// Divide the smoothie between two mason jars and serve.

1 to 1½ cups nondairy milk (such as almond, cashew, hemp, etc.)

1 frozen banana

2 tablespoons almond butter

1 scoop vegan vanilla protein powder

1 tablespoon pure maple syrup, or 1 or 2 pitted dates

⅔ cup canned pure pumpkin puree

2 teaspoons pumpkin pie spice

Pinch of sea salt

Ice cubes (about 1 cup)

PART
TWO

—

TIER 1
RECIPES

—

PAGE
199

APPLE PIE SMOOTHIE

SERVES

1

Here's America's favorite treat, whipped up in a decadent smoothie. Using just a few tasty ingredients, it's super easy to blend up for breakfast or for a snack.

// In a blender, combine the bananas, cashews, pecans, applesauce, dates, protein powder, nondairy milk, cinnamon, and nutmeg to taste and blend until smooth.

// Serve the smoothie in a mason jar, topped with apple slices, nuts, and a sprinkle of cinnamon.

2 frozen bananas

Handful of cashews, plus more for serving

Handful of pecans, plus more for serving

½ cup unsweetened applesauce

2 pitted dates (optional)

1 scoop vegan vanilla protein powder

1 cup nondairy milk (such as almond, cashew, hemp, etc.)

½ teaspoon ground cinnamon, plus more for garnish

Freshly grated nutmeg

Apple slices, for serving

BANANA-WALNUT OVERNIGHT OATS

SERVES
2

My family loves overnight oats—they're hearty, delicious, and super easy to make. Plus, because they can be prepared the night before, they make starting the day on a healthy note a lot easier. You can easily make this recipe in larger batches to be enjoyed throughout the week.

1 cup rolled oats

4 teaspoons chia seeds

1½ cups sweetened vanilla almond milk or other nondairy milk

1 large ripe banana, diced

¼ cup chopped raw walnuts

1 tablespoon pure maple syrup (optional)

// In a small bowl, stir together the oats, chia seeds, and almond milk.

// Refrigerate the mixture overnight, or for at least a few hours.

// When ready to serve, stir the oats and pour them into a mason jar. Top with the banana and walnuts.

// Drizzle the maple syrup over the top for an extra touch of natural sweetness, if desired.

PART
TWO

—

TIER 1
RECIPES

—

PAGE
201

HERBED WHITE BEAN AND PEA SALAD

SERVES
2

This salad is so delicious and easy to make. Keep it light and simple with a slice of multigrain toast or scoop it into romaine lettuce leaves. For a more filling meal, enjoy it with a side of cooked quinoa or brown rice. Make it your own.

// Put the frozen peas in a colander and set them under cool running water to thaw. Drain the peas well, then transfer them to a large bowl and add the beans, bell pepper, and scallion.

// TO MAKE THE DRESSING In a medium bowl, whisk together all the dressing ingredients and 2 tablespoons water. (Alternatively, combine the ingredients in a food processor and process until smooth.) Taste and adjust the seasoning, if necessary.

// Pour the dressing over the pea mixture and stir to combine.

// Top the salad with the sliced avocado. Season with a few grinds of black pepper and serve with your favorite fresh herbs sprinkled over the top.

1 cup frozen peas

1 (15-ounce) can butter beans or cannellini beans, drained and rinsed

½ red bell pepper, minced

1 scallion, thinly sliced

DRESSING

½ cup minced fresh mint

½ cup minced fresh parsley leaves

1 tablespoon minced fresh dill

1 teaspoon minced garlic

Juice of 1 lemon

¼ teaspoon sea salt

1 tablespoon extra-virgin olive oil

TO SERVE

1 avocado, sliced

Freshly ground black pepper

Fresh herbs (such as basil, thyme, and/or tarragon)

PART
TWO

—

TIER 1
RECIPES

—

PAGE
202

RAW BROCCOLI SALAD

SERVES
2

Broccoli is a detoxifying veggie and a great source of vitamins C and K, folate, potassium, and fiber. Broccoli also helps build skin-firming collagen and is brimming with antioxidants.

// In a large bowl, toss together the broccoli, tomatoes, bell pepper, pumpkin seeds, and red onion to combine.

// **TO MAKE THE DRESSING** In a small bowl, whisk together the mustard, vinegar, maple syrup, lemon juice, and 1 tablespoon water until smooth.

// Pour the dressing over the vegetables and toss to coat evenly, or drizzle over the top for a lighter coating. Leftover dressing can be stored in an airtight container in the refrigerator for up to 5 days.

6 cups chopped broccoli florets

2 cups cherry tomatoes, sliced

1 yellow bell pepper, chopped

1 cup hulled pumpkin seeds, toasted lightly until barely brown in a 350°F oven

½ cup finely chopped red onion

DRESSING

⅓ cup stone-ground mustard

¼ cup cider vinegar

2 teaspoons pure maple syrup

1 tablespoon fresh lemon juice

PART
TWO

—

TIER 1
RECIPES

—

PAGE
203

RAW VEGGIE SALAD

We love raw veggies in our home, and we especially love how they make us feel after we've enjoyed them as a meal. Here's a family favorite you're bound to enjoy as much as we do. It's loaded with health-boosting nutrients, not to mention flavor.

// TO MAKE THE DRESSING In a small bowl, whisk together all the dressing ingredients and 1 tablespoon water.

// TO MAKE THE SALAD In a large bowl, combine the cucumber, carrot, and broccoli.

// Pour the dressing over the veggies and toss to coat.

// Top with the olives, tomatoes, and pine nuts and serve.

TIP

Feel free to add any other veggies you have handy. This recipe is a great way to use up fresh produce that's languishing in your fridge.

DRESSING

⅓ cup stone-ground mustard

¼ cup cider vinegar

1 teaspoon pure maple syrup

¼ teaspoon freshly ground black pepper

1 tablespoon fresh lemon juice

SALAD

1 large cucumber, spiralized

1 large carrot, spiralized

1 large broccoli stem, tough outer layer peeled, spiralized

¼ cup pitted kalamata olives

1 cup cherry tomatoes, halved

¼ cup pine nuts

PART
TWO

—

TIER 1
RECIPES

—

PAGE

204

PREP: **15 MINUTES** / *COOK:* **0 MINUTES** / *TOTAL:* **15 MINUTES**

RAW RAINBOW SALAD

SERVES
2

This beautiful, colorful salad is made up of raw veggies that are loaded with vitamins, minerals, fiber, and antioxidants. It's perfect for lunch bowls or packed in mason jars for to-go meals.

// In a large bowl, combine all the salad ingredients.

// In a small bowl, whisk together all the dressing ingredients.

// Pour the dressing over the salad and toss to coat.

SALAD

1 head broccoli, finely chopped

1 orange bell pepper, finely chopped

1 red bell pepper, finely chopped

1 green bell pepper, finely chopped

4 small radishes, finely chopped

1 seedless (English) cucumber, finely chopped

¼ cup raw sunflower seeds

¼ cup raw hulled pumpkin seeds

DRESSING

¼ cup fresh lemon juice

1 tablespoon fresh orange juice

2 tablespoons extra-virgin olive oil

1 tablespoon Dijon mustard

½ teaspoon minced garlic

½ teaspoon sea salt

¼ teaspoon freshly ground black pepper

PART
TWO

—

TIER 1
RECIPES

—

PAGE
205

VEGAN MINESTRONE SOUP

SERVES
4

Minestrone soup—need I say more? Soups warm my soul. The base of this Italian favorite is tomatoes, which are brimming with antioxidants, vitamins C and K, potassium, and folate. Beans add the protein. Enjoy this hearty soup alone, with a side salad, or with a slice of your favorite toast.

// In a large pot, combine the broth and crushed tomatoes and bring to a boil.

// Add the chopped tomato, potato, squash, carrot, beans, and pasta. Add the cumin, coriander, paprika, basil, oregano, salt, pepper, and onion powder and stir to combine. Reduce the heat to low and simmer, stirring occasionally, for about 25 minutes.

// Taste and adjust the seasonings. If necessary, add water until the desired consistency is reached.

// Stir in the spinach and cook for 5 minutes more.

// Ladle into bowls, garnish with fresh herbs, if desired, and serve.

4 cups vegetable broth

1½ cups organic crushed tomatoes, strained

1 small tomato, cored and chopped

1 small Yukon Gold potato, cubed

1 yellow squash, cubed

1 large carrot, sliced

1 (15-ounce) can cannellini beans, drained and rinsed

1 cup gluten-free pasta, any shape

2 teaspoons ground cumin

2 teaspoons ground coriander

1 teaspoon paprika

½ teaspoon dried basil

½ teaspoon dried oregano

½ teaspoon sea salt

½ teaspoon freshly ground black pepper

¼ teaspoon onion powder

1 cup chopped spinach or stemmed kale leaves

Fresh herbs, for garnish (optional)

PART
TWO

—

TIER 1
RECIPES

—

PAGE
206

MAGGIE'S SPICY EGGPLANT STIR-FRY

SERVES

4

You will never miss chicken, beef, or seafood in a stir-fry after you make this dish. Eggplant is a versatile veggie because it matches up, tastewise, to any cuisine in which it is used. Here it performs like a charm and lends a "meaty" flavor to a classic Asian stir-fry.

// TO MAKE THE SAUCE In a small bowl, whisk together all the sauce ingredients and ¼ cup water until smooth. Set aside.

// TO MAKE THE STIR-FRY In a large skillet, heat the olive oil over medium-high heat. Add the eggplant and cook, stirring, for 3 minutes. Add 1 cup water and cover the pan. Cook for 5 minutes, or until eggplant has softened.

// Uncover the pan and stir in the garlic, onion, spinach, and bell pepper. Cover and cook until all veggies are just soft, about 7 minutes.

// Uncover the pan, stir in the sauce, and cook until the sauce has thickened.

// Serve the stir-fry over riced cauliflower, quinoa, or brown rice, garnished with the cashews.

SAUCE

½ cup coconut aminos

2 tablespoons agave nectar

2 tablespoons hot sauce or sriracha

1 tablespoon cornstarch

STIR-FRY

¼ cup olive oil

1 medium eggplant, peeled and cubed

6 garlic cloves, minced

1 medium onion, chopped

2 handfuls of fresh spinach, torn

1 red bell pepper, chopped

Riced cauliflower, cooked quinoa, or cooked brown rice, for serving

½ cup chopped raw cashews, for topping

AVOCADO AND BROCCOLI LETTUCE CUPS

SERVES
2

Here's a quick and easy way to add more greens to your diet. Broccoli is a super source of vitamins A, B, C, E, and K, folate, fiber, potassium, and phenolic compounds that help protect against cancer, diabetes, and heart disease. The avocado and cherry tomatoes give it an added nutritional burst.

// Set a steamer basket in a medium saucepan and add water to come just below the bottom of the basket. Bring the water to a simmer over medium heat. Put the broccoli in the steamer, cover, and cook for 5 minutes, or until tender.

// Transfer the broccoli to a large bowl. Add the tomatoes, avocado, lime juice, and pepper and toss to combine.

// Spoon the broccoli mixture into the lettuce leaves, top with the nutritional yeast, and serve.

1 head broccoli, chopped

1 cup cherry tomatoes, sliced

½ Hass avocado, cut into small cubes

Juice of ½ lime

Pinch of freshly ground black pepper

1 head butter lettuce, leaves separated

2 tablespoons nutritional yeast

TIP

For added crunch, top with fresh sprouts and/or seeds.

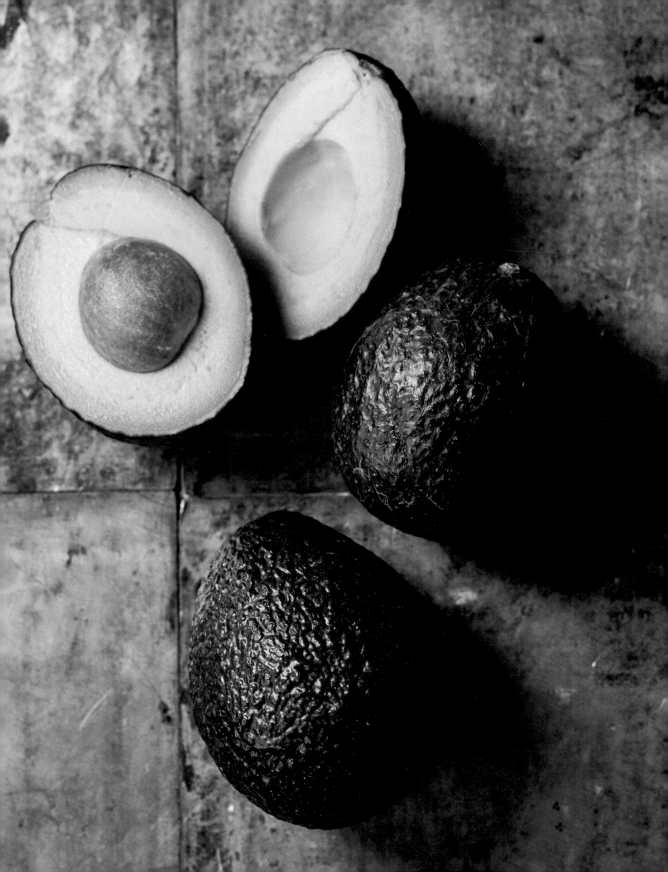

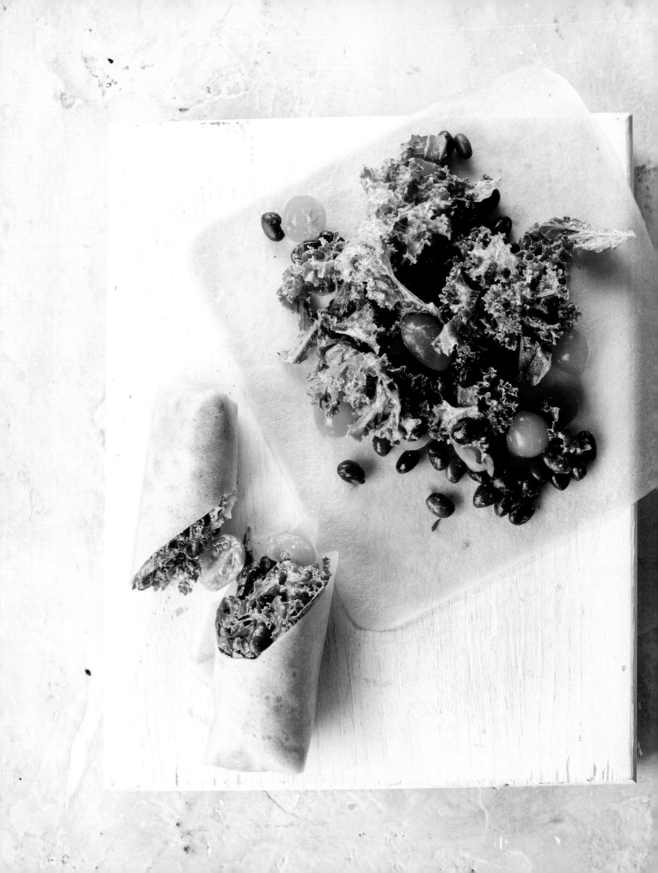

BLACK BEAN AND KALE WRAP

SERVES
2

Black beans and kale are nutritious enough on their own, but when they come together, they form a perfect meal that is loaded with vitamins, minerals, protein, and fiber. Here's a way to do that in a simple-to-prepare wrap.

// TO MAKE THE DRESSING Put the cashews in a small bowl and add warm or hot filtered water to cover. Set aside to soak overnight.

// Drain and rinse the cashews and transfer them to a food processor. Add the nutritional yeast, lime juice, and 1/2 cup water and process until the dressing is smooth.

// In a medium bowl, combine the kale and 1/4 cup of the dressing. Using clean hands, massage the dressing into the kale to soften the leaves.

// In small saucepan, heat the black beans over moderate heat until warmed through.

// Divide the kale, beans, and tomatoes between the coconut wraps, drizzle more dressing over top, and fold to enclose the filling. Serve immediately.

DRESSING

½ cup raw cashews

2 tablespoons nutritional yeast

2 tablespoons fresh lime juice

3 cups stemmed and chopped kale leaves

2 cups cooked or canned black beans, drained and rinsed, if canned

1 cup cherry tomatoes, sliced

2 coconut wraps (this is a healthy, gluten-free, low-carb, and vegan alternative to tortillas, available in whole-foods stores or through retailers such as Amazon)

TIP

If you're pressed for time, skip the overnight soaking and instead soak the cashews in warm filtered water for just a few minutes. Drain and rinse as directed.

PART
TWO

—

TIER 1
RECIPES

—

PAGE

211

PEANUT BUTTER SMOOTHIE BOWL

SERVES
1

Smoothie bowls are a fun way to start the day, especially when they're as delicious and nutritious as this one!

// In a blender, combine the frozen banana, almond milk, and peanut butter and blend until smooth.

// Scoop the smoothie into a bowl and top with the sliced banana and peanuts. Garnish with fresh berries for a little extra color and an added antioxidant boost.

1½ ripe bananas: 1 frozen, ½ sliced

½ cup almond milk or other nondairy milk

2 tablespoons peanut butter

2 tablespoons raw peanuts

Fresh berries

PART
TWO

—

TIER 2
RECIPES

—

PAGE
212

HOMEMADE GRANOLA

SERVES
5

This nut-free granola is a perfect on-the-go, protein-rich breakfast or snack. Plus it's made with only four simple ingredients.

3 cups rolled oats

½ cup raw sunflower seeds

½ cup raw hulled pumpkin seeds

⅓ cup pure maple syrup

// Preheat the oven to 325ºF.

// In a large bowl, combine all the ingredients and mix until the oats and seeds are evenly coated with the syrup.

// Spread the mixture evenly over a large baking sheet and bake for 20 to 25 minutes, until golden brown.

// Let cool, then store in an airtight container at room temperature for up to 2 weeks.

PART
TWO

—

TIER 2
RECIPES

—

PAGE
213

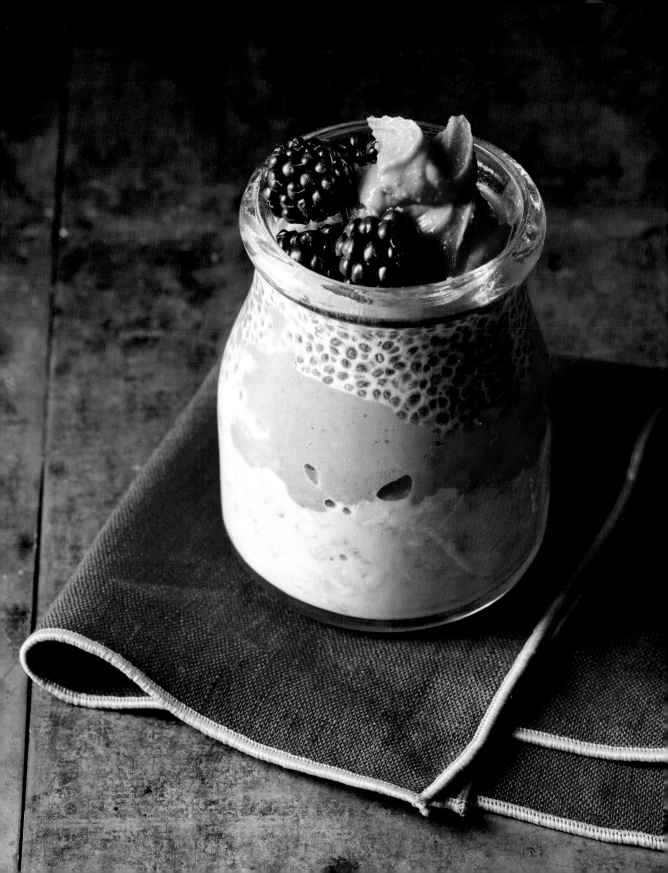

CHIA OAT PEANUT BUTTER PARFAIT

SERVES
2

This parfait is a nutritious and easy make-ahead breakfast. The delicious combination of oats, chia, blackberries, and peanut butter is a great way to fuel your day!

// In a mason jar or other glass container with a lid, stir together the chia seeds, 1 cup of the almond milk, and the maple syrup.

// In a separate jar or other glass container with a lid, stir together the oats and remaining 1 cup almond milk.

// Cover both jars and refrigerate overnight.

// When ready to enjoy, stir the oat and chia mixtures to make sure each mixture is well combined and to break apart any clumps.

// In a serving jar, layer half the oat mixture, 1 tablespoon of the peanut butter, and half the chia pudding. Top with 1 tablespoon more peanut butter and 2 tablespoons of the blackberries. Repeat the layers in a second jar using the remaining ingredients and serve.

3 tablespoons chia seeds

2 cups unsweetened vanilla almond milk

1 teaspoon pure maple syrup

½ cup rolled oats

4 tablespoons peanut butter

4 tablespoons blackberries

BLUEBERRY BLISS BOWL

SERVES
1

Smoothie bowls are a quick and easy way to enjoy a nutritious and delicious breakfast that provides the energy you'll need to get your day going. This one is loaded with antioxidant power!

// In a blender, combine the frozen banana, 1/2 cup of the blueberries, chia seeds, and almond milk and blend until smooth.

// Serve the smoothie in a bowl, topped with the remaining 1/2 cup blueberries, the blackberries, and the sliced banana.

1½ ripe bananas: 1 frozen and ½ sliced

1 cup frozen blueberries

1 tablespoon ground chia seeds

½ cup almond milk or other nondairy milk

½ cup fresh blackberries

TIP

Feel free to get creative with different fruit and seed toppings.

HEARTS OF PALM AND SWEET PEA PASTA SALAD

SERVES
2

This pasta salad is delicious and easy to make. The nutritious combination of hearts of palm, sweet peas, tomato, parsley, avocado, capers, and nutritional yeast is loaded with vitamins and minerals.

// Bring a large pot of water to a boil. Add the pasta and cook according to the package instructions. Drain and transfer to a large bowl.

// Add the olive oil, lime juice, parsley, tomatoes, avocado, hearts of palm, peas, capers, and nutritional yeast and toss to combine.

// Season with salt and pepper and serve.

1 cup uncooked pasta, any shape

2 tablespoons olive oil

Juice of 1 lime

Leaves from ½ bunch parsley, minced

8 cherry tomatoes, quartered

½ Hass avocado, sliced

4 pieces canned hearts of palm, drained and sliced

1 cup canned sweet peas, drained and rinsed

2 teaspoons capers

2 tablespoons nutritional yeast

Sea salt and freshly ground black pepper

PART
TWO

—

TIER 2
RECIPES

—

PAGE
217

AVOCADO TOAST WITH SUNFLOWER SEEDS AND SPROUTS

SERVES
1

This is an all-time family favorite. I fix it most days of the week for my kids. Avocados are incredibly nutritious and contain a wide variety of vitamins and minerals—they even have more potassium than bananas. They're also loaded with fiber and contain heart-healthy monounsaturated fats. Avocado, however, isn't the only superstar in this recipe. The sunflower seeds and sprouts make this a perfect meal, any time of day.

2 slices gluten-free vegan bread

½ Hass avocado

Juice of ½ lime

1 tablespoon raw sunflower seeds

½ cup broccoli sprouts

Dash of smoked paprika

// Toast the bread.

// In a small bowl, use a fork to mash the avocado with the lime juice.

// Spread the mashed avocado over the toast. Top with the sunflower seeds, sprouts, and paprika and serve.

PART
TWO

—

TIER 2
RECIPES

—

PAGE
218

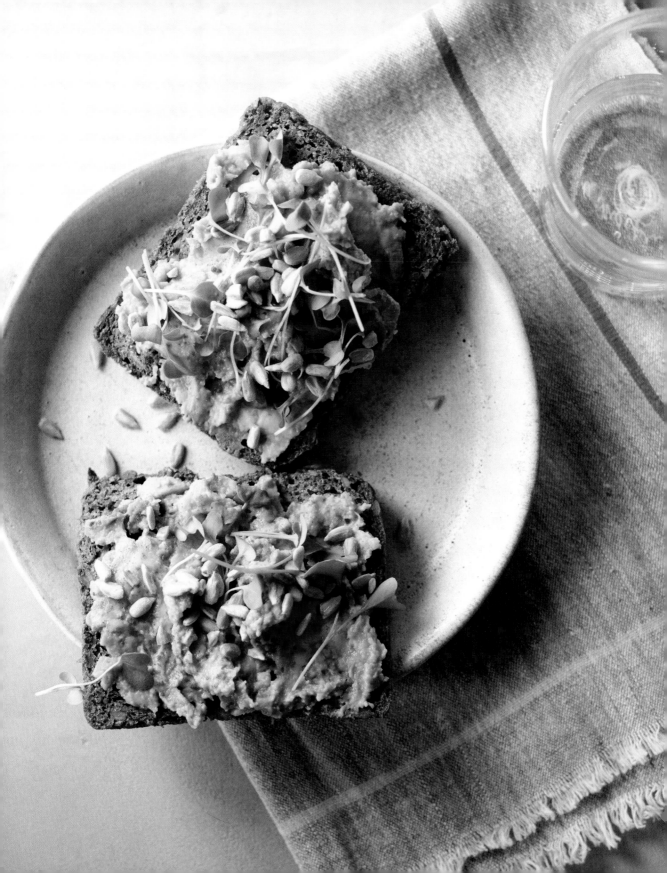

SHREDDED BRUSSELS SPROUTS SALAD

SERVES
4

Brussels sprouts are low in calories but loaded with vitamins, minerals, and fiber. This simple and easy-to-make salad will help reduce inflammation while protecting you against certain types of cancer. It's crunchy and scrumptious, too.

// Set a steamer basket in a medium saucepan and add water to come just below the bottom of the basket. Bring the water to a simmer over medium heat. Put the peas in the steamer, cover, and cook for a few minutes, until tender.

// Meanwhile, in a large bowl, combine the Brussels sprouts, carrots, and cabbage. Add the peas and almonds and toss to combine.

// **TO MAKE THE DRESSING** In a small bowl, combine all the dressing ingredients and whisk until smooth.

// Pour the dressing over the vegetables and toss to coat. Serve immediately.

1 cup frozen peas

6 cups shaved Brussels sprouts

2 cups grated carrots

2 cups shredded cabbage

½ cup raw almonds

DRESSING

¼ cup coconut aminos

2 tablespoons peanut butter

2 tablespoons fresh lime juice

1 teaspoon grated fresh ginger

1 tablespoon pure maple syrup

TIP

If you're planning on saving some of the salad for leftovers, set that portion aside before adding the dressing, and store the salad and dressing separately until ready to serve.

PART
TWO

—

TIER 2
RECIPES

—

PAGE
220

SWEET POTATO TOAST WITH HUMMUS AND BROCCOLI SPROUTS

SERVES
2

Slicing and roasting (or toasting) sweet potato makes it a delicious bread replacement. The hummus adds a protein boost.

1 sweet potato, cut into ¼-inch-thick slices

1 cup hummus, store-bought or homemade (page 284)

1 (8-ounce) container broccoli sprouts

// Preheat the oven to 350°F.

// Arrange the sweet potato slices in a single layer on a baking sheet. Bake until the slices are tender, about 20 minutes. (You can also cook these in a toaster, but you may need to run the toaster on high for three or four cycles.)

// Top each sweet potato slice with some of the hummus and sprouts, and serve. Store any leftover sweet potato slices, without toppings, in an airtight container in the refrigerator for up to 1 week. Reheat in the toaster or toaster oven and top as directed.

PART
TWO

—

TIER 2
RECIPES

—

PAGE
221

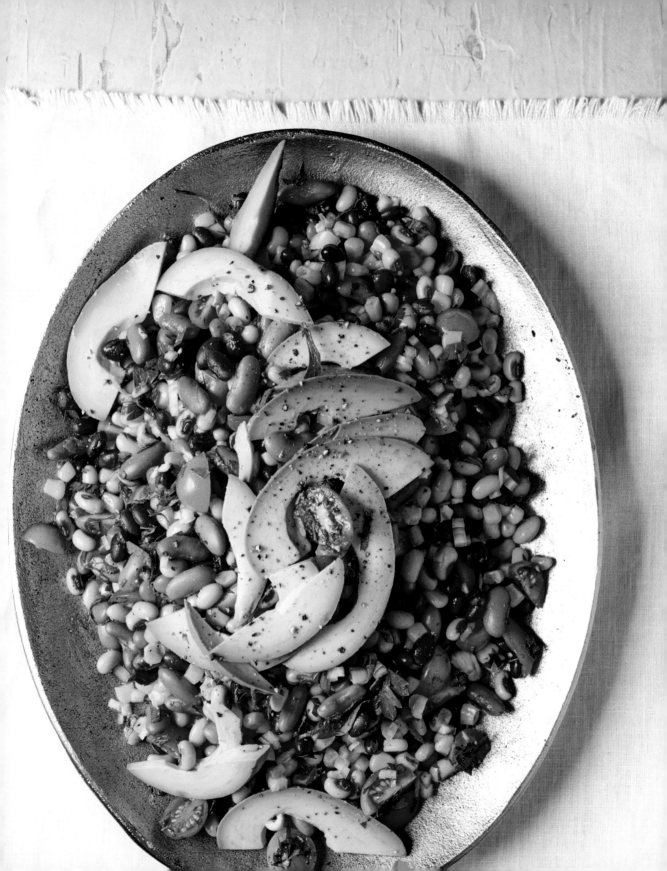

MEXICAN-INSPIRED BEAN SALAD

SERVES
2

This delicious salad is made with a nutritious combination of plant superstars, all mixed together in a citrus dressing and topped with sliced avocado. If your kids will be enjoying this salad and are sensitive to spicy foods, you can skip the chili powder. If not, for a more authentic Mexican experience, feel free to add minced jalapeños for added kick, and use cilantro instead of parsley.

// In a large bowl, combine the black-eyed peas, pinto beans, black beans, and corn. Add the tomatoes, onion, parsley, lemon juice, olive oil (if using), vinegar, salt, pepper, and chili powder (if using). Mix together to combine. Taste and adjust the seasoning if necessary.

// Top with the avocado, season with salt and pepper, and serve.

1 (15-ounce) can black-eyed peas, drained and rinsed

1 (15-ounce) can pinto beans, drained and rinsed

1 (15-ounce) can black beans, drained and rinsed

1 (15-ounce) can corn, drained and rinsed

1 cup cherry tomatoes, quartered

⅓ red onion, minced

Leaves from ½ bunch parsley or cilantro, minced (about ¾ cup)

Juice of 2 lemons

1 tablespoon olive oil (optional)

1 tablespoon red wine vinegar

½ teaspoon sea salt, plus more as needed

¼ teaspoon freshly ground black pepper, plus more as needed

¼ teaspoon chili powder, or to taste (optional)

1 avocado, sliced

PART
TWO

———

TIER 2
RECIPES

———

PAGE
223

SPLIT PEA SOUP

SERVES
4

As a kid, one of my favorite meals was split pea soup. Not much has changed since then. Split peas are an amazing source of protein, fiber, iron, calcium, magnesium, and manganese. They're known for reducing risk of cancer, regulating blood sugar levels, lowering cholesterol, and improving heart health. I loved them before I knew anything about their benefits, and now I eat them all the time.

// In a large pot, combine the split peas, paprika, cumin, garlic, potatoes, carrot, onion, lemon juice, and pepper. Add 8 cups water and bring to a boil. Reduce the heat to low and simmer for 30 to 40 minutes, until the peas are tender.

// Ladle into bowls, garnish with parsley, and serve.

2 cups dried split peas, soaked overnight in filtered water

1 tablespoon smoked paprika

2 tablespoons ground cumin

1 teaspoon minced garlic

4 small potatoes, cubed

1 large carrot, diced

½ small onion, diced

Juice of 1 lemon

¼ teaspoon freshly ground black pepper

Chopped fresh parsley, for garnish

TIP

This dish can be enjoyed with quinoa or brown rice for a heartier meal.

PART
TWO

—

TIER 2
RECIPES

—

PAGE
224

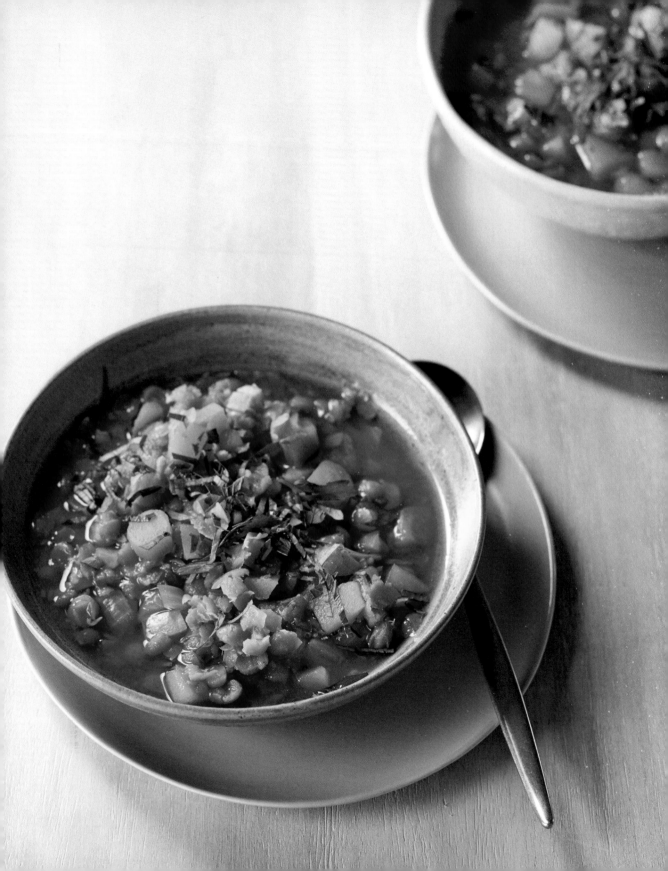

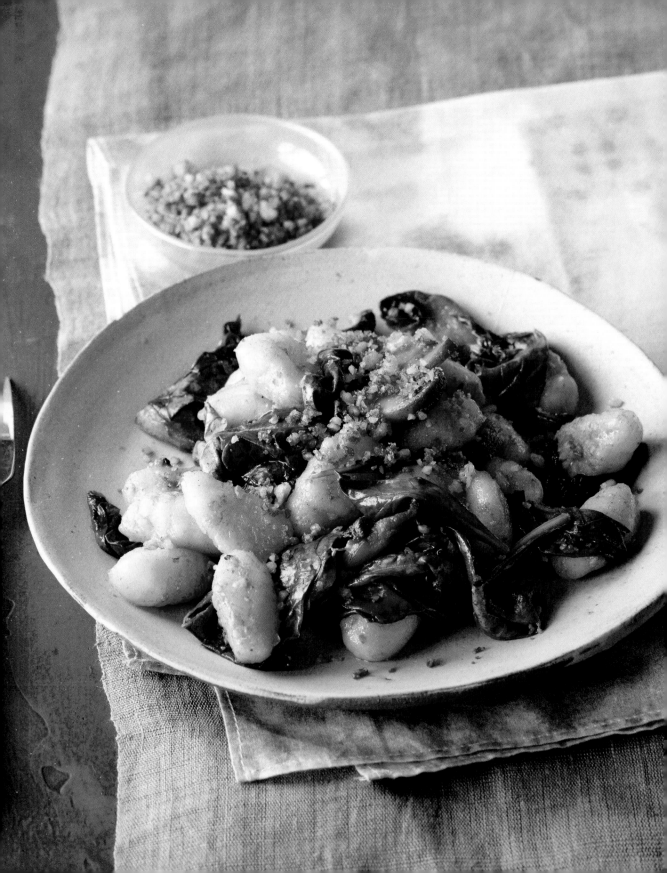

SPINACH AND MUSHROOM GNOCCHI WITH WALNUT MEAT

SERVES
2

Gnocchi is a potato-based pasta that is super healthy thanks to its heart-friendly potassium. It therefore makes a great foundation for a delicious plant-based meal. This is my all-time favorite gnocchi dish! You'll be amazed by how simple it is to make, and you'll instantly fall in love with its rich flavors and textures.

// Bring a large pot of water to a boil.

// **TO MAKE THE WALNUT MEAT** In a food processor, combine the walnuts, vinegar, coconut aminos, cumin, coriander, and paprika. Season with garlic powder and pepper. Pulse several times until the walnuts are broken down and crumbly, making sure not to overprocess the mixture into a paste. Set aside.

// Add the gnocchi to the boiling water and cook until they float to the top. Drain and set aside.

// In a medium skillet, heat the olive oil over medium-high heat. Add the mushrooms and cook, stirring, for a few minutes, until browned. Reduce the heat to medium, add the gnocchi and most of the walnut meat (reserving some for garnish), and cook, stirring gently, for a few more minutes.

// Toss in the spinach and stir until wilted.

// Serve the gnocchi garnished with the reserved walnut meat.

WALNUT MEAT

¼ cup raw walnuts

1 teaspoon balsamic vinegar

½ teaspoon coconut aminos

1 teaspoon ground cumin

1 teaspoon ground coriander

Pinch of smoked paprika

Garlic powder

Freshly ground black pepper

1½ cups store-bought gnocchi (choose a brand made without eggs)

2 tablespoons olive oil

1 cup sliced fresh button mushrooms

1 cup fresh spinach

LOADED SWEET POTATO

SERVES
2

Every bite of this meal is bursting with flavor: the perfect combination of sweet-and-savory sweet potato with sautéed black beans and kale, and the creaminess of the cashew dressing.

// Put the cashews in a small bowl, add warm or hot filtered water to cover, and set aside to soak for 2 to 3 hours.

// Preheat the oven to 400°F. Line a baking sheet with parchment paper.

// Place the sweet potatoes on the prepared baking sheet and prick them several times with a fork. Roast for 45 minutes to 1 hour, until fork-tender (the cooking time will vary based on the size of the potato). (Alternatively, to reduce the cooking time, slice the potatoes in half lengthwise, place them cut-side down on the baking sheet, and roast for 30 to 35 minutes.)

// In a large skillet, heat the olive oil over medium heat. Add the black beans, kale, and a pinch of salt and cook, stirring occasionally, until the kale has wilted and the beans are warmed through. Keep warm.

// Drain the cashews and transfer them to a food processor or high-speed blender. Add the nutritional yeast, lemon juice, $1/4$ teaspoon salt, and 3 tablespoons water and blend until smooth.

// Gently slice each roasted sweet potato lengthwise. Using a fork, mash some of the flesh.

// Top the sweet potatoes evenly with the black bean mixture and the avocado. Drizzle with the cashew dressing and season with pepper. Garnish with chives and serve.

3 tablespoons raw cashews

2 medium sweet potatoes

1 tablespoon olive oil

1 (15-ounce) can black beans, drained and rinsed

1 cup chopped stemmed kale leaves

¼ teaspoon sea salt, plus more as needed

1 tablespoon nutritional yeast

Juice of ½ lemon

½ avocado, sliced

Freshly ground black pepper

Minced fresh chives, for garnish

TIP

I recommend making a larger batch of the dressing to store in an airtight container in the fridge and enjoy throughout the week in other recipes. Also, when you're using a high-speed blender, it can be easier to blend larger quantities of ingredients.

PART
TWO

—

TIER 2
RECIPES

—

PAGE
228

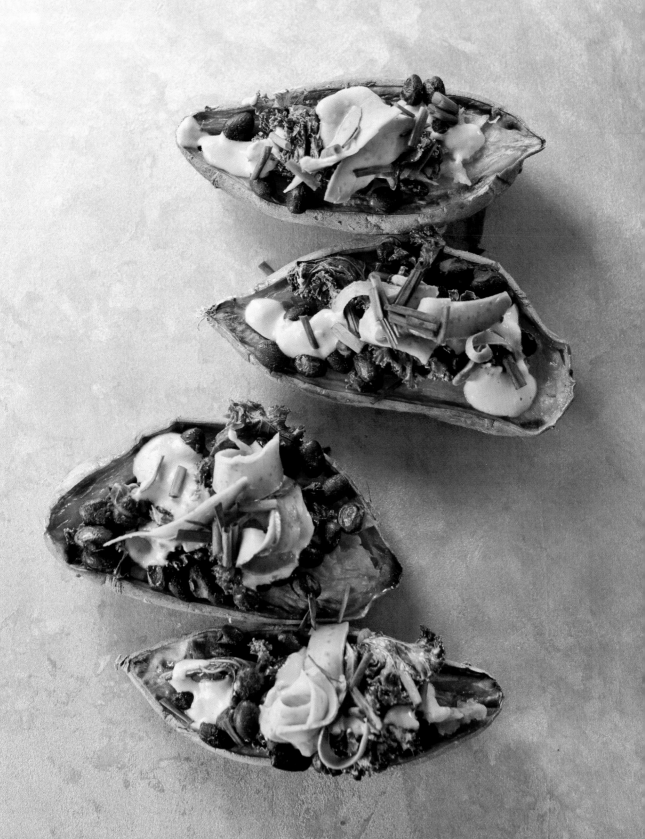

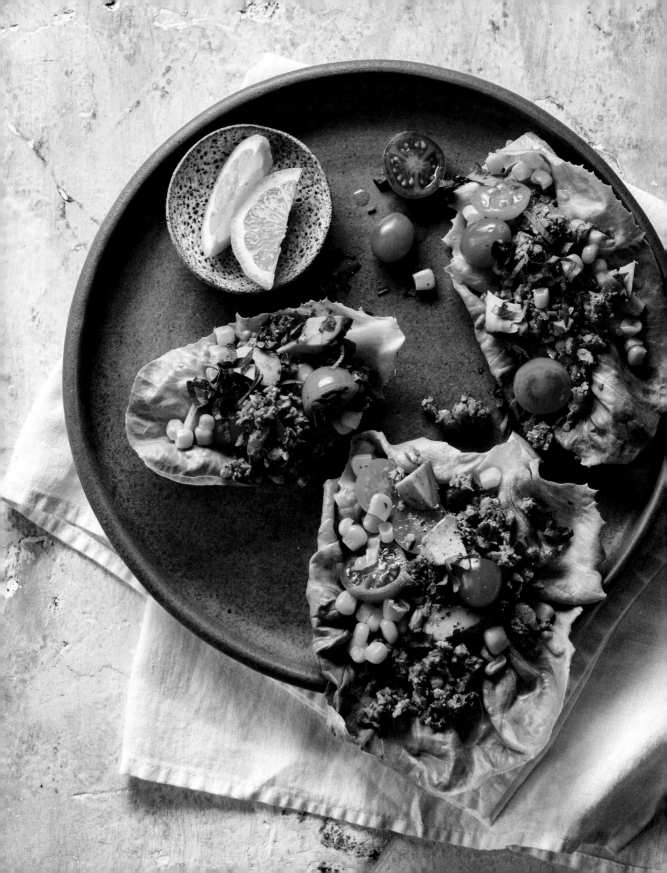

MUSHROOM "CHORIZO" LETTUCE TACOS

SERVES
4

These lettuce tacos are a family favorite in our home, and I'm sure they'll be in yours, too. Keep in mind, when making this recipe, you might want to make an extra batch of the mushroom "chorizo," and store in the fridge to enjoy with other recipes, like we do. It adds great flavor and a nutritional boost to any meal.

// TO MAKE THE MUSHROOM "CHORIZO" In a food processor, combine all the chorizo ingredients and pulse until crumbly, stopping to scrape down the sides several times.

// Heat a large skillet over medium heat. Add the chorizo and cook, stirring frequently to prevent burning, for about 5 minutes, or until browned and cooked through. Remove from the heat.

// Spoon the chorizo into the lettuce cups. Top with the corn, tomatoes, and avocado and garnish with parsley. Serve with the lemon wedges alongside for squeezing over the top.

MUSHROOM "CHORIZO"

1 cup sliced mushrooms, any type

¾ cup raw walnuts

6 jarred sun-dried tomatoes in olive oil

½ teaspoon minced garlic

1 teaspoon ground cumin

½ teaspoon smoked paprika

¼ teaspoon freshly ground black pepper

Pinch of cayenne pepper

½ teaspoon sea salt

1 head butter lettuce, leaves separated and stemmed

½ cup canned corn kernels, drained and rinsed

¼ cup cherry tomatoes, quartered

½ avocado, sliced

Minced fresh parsley, for garnish

Lemon wedges, for serving

PART
TWO

TIER 2
RECIPES

PAGE
231

CHICKPEA NO-TUNA SALAD SANDWICH

SERVES
2

Introducing another family favorite: "no-tuna" salad made with chickpeas. We make this a couple of times a week and enjoy it in a sandwich, with sliced carrots and celery sticks, as a dip for gluten-free crackers, or in a generous scoop atop a green salad.

// In a medium bowl, mash the chickpeas with a fork or the bottom of a cup until broken down to a creamy but still slightly chunky consistency. Add the carrot, onion, parsley, mayo, mustard, garlic powder, lemon juice, salt, and pepper to taste. Mix well to combine. Taste and adjust the seasoning if necessary.

// Divide the lettuce, tomato, and no-tuna salad between 2 slices of the bread, then top each with a second slice of bread and serve.

TIP

Make a large batch of no-tuna salad to have on hand throughout the week and store it in an airtight container in the fridge for up to 5 days.

1 (15-ounce) can chickpeas, drained and rinsed, loose skins discarded

2 tablespoons shredded carrot

2 tablespoons minced red onion

2 tablespoons minced fresh parsley, or 1 tablespoon dried

2 tablespoons vegan mayo

1 teaspoon Dijon mustard

Pinch of garlic powder

Juice of ½ lemon

⅛ teaspoon sea salt, or to taste

Freshly ground black pepper

Lettuce or other greens

½ tomato, sliced

4 slices gluten-free vegan bread

PART
TWO

—

TIER 2
RECIPES

—

PAGE
232

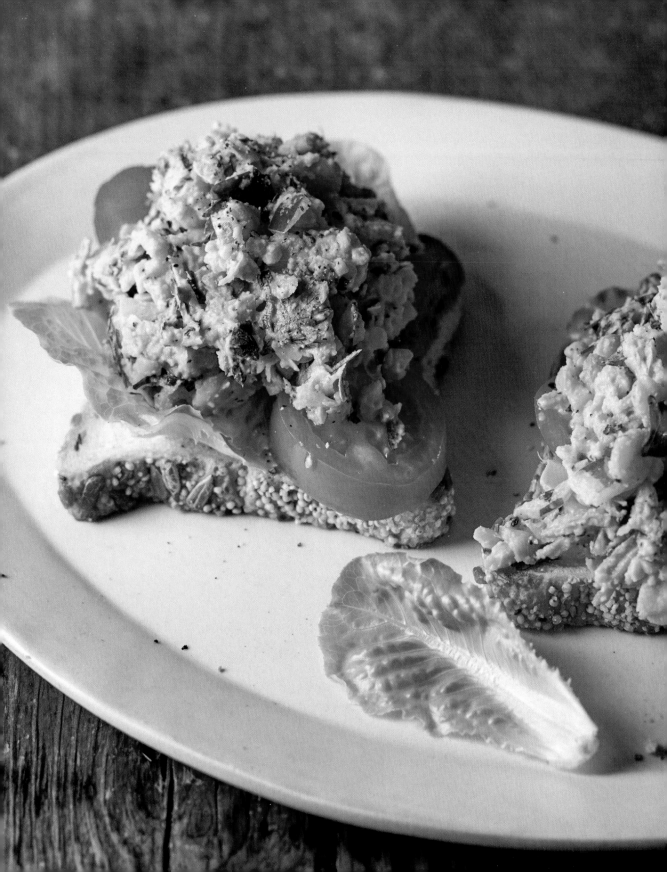

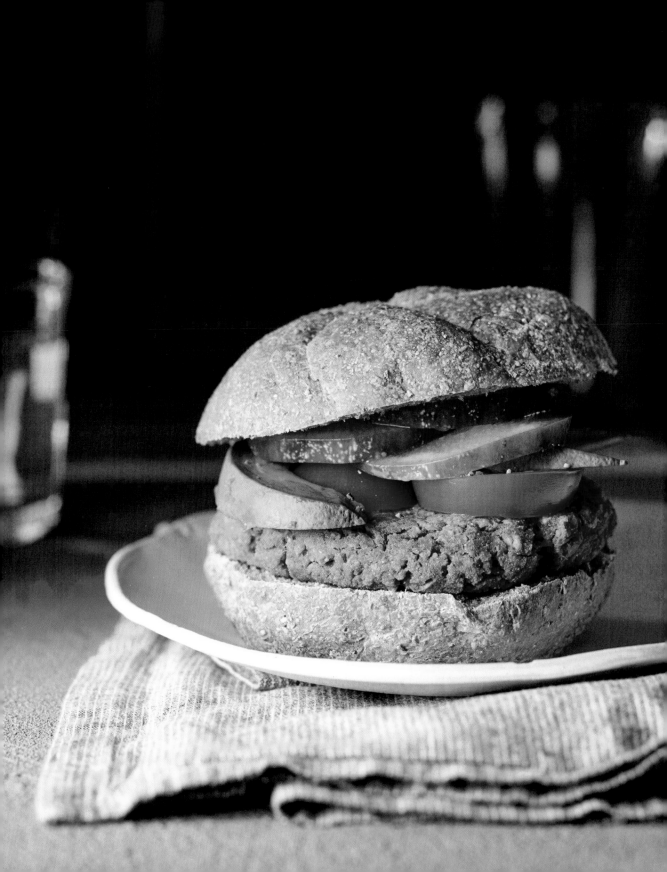

CHICKPEA AND AVOCADO BURGERS

SERVES 4

Veggie burgers are both delicious and nutritious. This simple chickpea burger, blended with sweet potato, is loaded with flavor and makes a perfect lunch or dinner.

// Preheat the oven to 400°F. Line a baking sheet with parchment paper.

// Place the sweet potato on the prepared baking sheet and prick it several times with a fork. Roast for 45 minutes to 1 hour, or until fork tender. Set aside until cool enough to handle, then peel the sweet potato and put the flesh in a large bowl.

// Add the chickpeas, chickpea flour, cumin, paprika, salt, and chili powder to the bowl and mash until all the ingredients are well incorporated. Cover and refrigerate for 30 minutes, or until the mixture firms up.

// **TO MAKE THE BURGERS** Preheat the oven to 400°F.

// Using your hands, form the sweet potato mixture into 4 patties and place them on a baking sheet. Bake for 30 to 40 minutes, flipping halfway through, until noticeably golden and crisp.

// Place the burgers on the buns and top with avocado, tomato, and pickles. Store any leftover burgers in an airtight container in the fridge for up to a few days or in the freezer for about 1 month.

BURGERS

1 large sweet potato

1½ cups canned chickpeas, drained, rinsed, and mashed

¼ cup chickpea flour

2 teaspoons ground cumin

2 teaspoons smoked paprika

½ teaspoon sea salt

½ teaspoon chili powder

4 whole-grain burger buns

1 avocado, sliced

1 small tomato, sliced

Pickle slices

PART
TWO

—

TIER 2
RECIPES

—

PAGE
235

BANANA-NUT QUINOA BOWL

SERVES
3

I love keeping cooked quinoa in the refrigerator for easy lunch bowls. Here I use it for a delicious and hearty breakfast that is sure to warm your heart. Quinoa is a great source of complete protein. When combined with banana, blueberries, and walnuts, it makes a perfect breakfast for the entire family.

// In a small saucepan, combine the quinoa and almond milk and cook over medium heat until the quinoa has absorbed the liquid.

// Pour the cooked quinoa into a small bowl and top with the banana, walnuts, and blueberries.

// Drizzle some almond butter over the top, if desired, and enjoy.

2 cups cooked quinoa (recipe follows)

¾ cup unsweetened vanilla almond milk or other nondairy milk

1 banana, sliced

⅓ cup chopped raw walnuts

½ cup blueberries

1 tablespoon almond butter (optional)

TIP

This is a very versatile dish and can be enjoyed with a variety of fruit (fresh or dried) and nut butters.

PART
TWO

—

TIER 3
RECIPES

—

PAGE
236

HOW TO COOK QUINOA

Quinoa has been enjoyed for thousands of years but recently has become one of the world's most popular superfoods. It's one of those foods that, by itself, can be a complete meal. It contains all the essential amino acids and is therefore a great source of protein. Quinoa is high in fiber, vitamins, minerals, and antioxidants and is naturally gluten-free. It's a staple in our home, and a container of cooked quinoa can always be found in our refrigerator, ready to enjoy in salads, quick bowls, and healthy snacks.

1 cup uncooked quinoa

// Rinse the quinoa in a fine-mesh colander and drain well.

// In a medium saucepan, combine the quinoa and 2 cups water and bring the water to a boil. Reduce the heat to medium-low, cover, and simmer for 12 to 15 minutes, until the water has been absorbed.

// Set aside, covered, for 5 minutes. Uncover and fluff the quinoa with a fork.

// Serve or let cool and store in an airtight container in the fridge for up to 1 week.

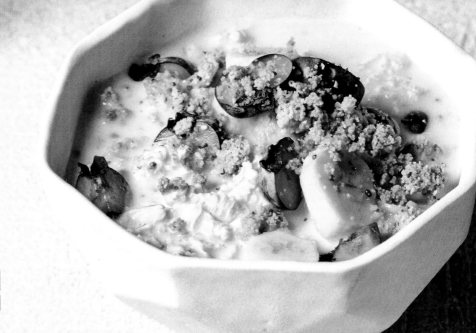

SERVES
2

PREP: **5 MINUTES** (plus overnight soaking) /
COOK: **10 MINUTES** / TOTAL: **15 MINUTES**

ALMOND GRANOLA OAT CUP

Start your day with this easy and delicious breakfast! Simply top the overnight oats with freshly baked almond granola, sliced banana, and blueberries.

// In a mason jar or other glass container with a lid, stir together the oats and almond milk. Cover and refrigerate overnight.

// When ready to enjoy, preheat the oven to 350°F. Line a baking sheet with parchment paper.

// In a medium bowl, combine the almond flour, chia seeds, and maple syrup and stir until crumbly. Transfer the almond granola mixture to the prepared baking sheet and bake for 8 to 10 minutes, until lightly golden.

// Divide the overnight oats between two bowls. Top with the almond granola, banana, and blueberries and enjoy!

1 cup rolled oats

1½ cups unsweetened vanilla almond milk

¼ cup plus 2 tablespoons almond flour

2 teaspoons ground chia seeds

1 tablespoon pure maple syrup

1 banana, sliced

½ cup blueberries

HOMEMADE OAT MILK

MAKES
4
CUPS

I love preparing my own dairy-alternative drinks at home. They're easy to make and less expensive than commercial varieties. What's more, making grain milks and nut milks at home lets you be in control of the ingredients that go into them. This oat milk recipe is nut-free and ready in 5 minutes or less. Plus, it's smooth and delicious, the perfect nondairy milk.

1 cup uncooked steel-cut oats

6 pitted dates, or more to taste

½ teaspoon pure vanilla extract

// In a high-speed blender, combine the oats, dates, vanilla, and 4 cups of filtered water and blend on high speed until smooth.

// Strain the oat milk through a nut milk bag or a fine-mesh sieve lined with cheesecloth into a large mason jar.

// Store the oat milk in the refrigerator, covered, for 4 to 5 days. Separation is natural—just shake thoroughly to recombine before using. Enjoy it in smoothies or overnight oats and with granola.

DRIED FRUIT BROWN RICE PORRIDGE

SERVES
2

A hearty, warm breakfast is always satisfying. Here's a quick and easy way to make one, especially if you have some leftover brown rice in your fridge.

// In a small saucepan, stir together the brown rice, almond milk, chia seeds, flaxseed, and dried cranberries. Cook over medium heat until thickened, about 10 minutes.

// Divide the porridge between two bowls and top with the blueberries, raspberries, and cashews. Serve warm.

2 cups cooked brown rice

1¼ cups unsweetened vanilla almond milk

1½ teaspoons ground chia seeds

1½ teaspoons ground flaxseed

2 tablespoons dried cranberries

½ cup blueberries

½ cup raspberries

¼ cup raw cashews

TIP

Reheat leftovers on the stovetop with a splash of almond milk or water.

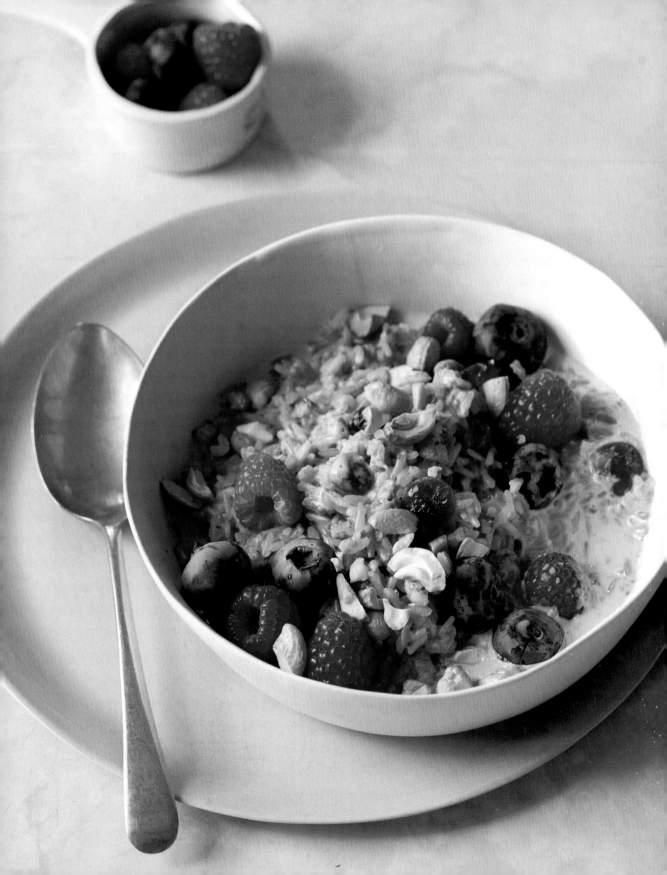

Almond milk is delicious and chock-full of healthy nutrients—but like many healthy foods, it can lose some of its nutritional power when it is produced for mass consumption. Almond milk can be used in pretty much any recipe that calls for regular milk—baked goods, soups, sauces, ice cream, or desserts—and it's absolutely delicious on its own! If you love almond milk and want to get the most nutrition, try making your own. It's really simple.

MAKE YOUR OWN

ALMOND MILK

///////

IT'S EASY!

1 cup raw almonds

1 tablespoon pure maple syrup

1 teaspoon pure vanilla extract

// Put the almonds in a medium bowl, add filtered water to cover, and set aside at a room temperature to soak 8 to 12 hours, or overnight.

// Drain and rinse the almonds, then dry them thoroughly and transfer them to a high-speed blender or food processor. Add the maple syrup, vanilla, and 3 cups water and blend until reasonably smooth.

// Strain the almond milk through a nut milk bag or a fine-mesh sieve lined with cheesecloth into a large mason jar. (Save the almond pulp to reuse in other recipes. See below.)

// Store the almond milk in the refrigerator, covered, for 2 to 3 days.

ALMOND PULP

The leftover almond pulp (also known as almond meal) can be used in smoothies, incorporated into baked goods, or mixed into yogurt or oatmeal. If you're not going to use the almond pulp immediately, dry it out or freeze it for later use. To dry the pulp into almond meal, use a dehydrator, or spread it over a parchment-lined baking sheet and bake in a preheated 200°F oven until completely dry (this might take a few hours). Store in the refrigerator for up to one week. To freeze almond pulp, pack in a freezable container for up to 1 month.

PREPARATION TIPS

Always opt for organic ingredients when possible.

Use filtered water for soaking and blending the almonds.

If you plan on making almond milk often, consider purchasing a reusable nut milk bag to strain out the pulp.

KALE BREAKFAST SALAD

SERVES

2

Kale for breakfast? You bet! There's no better way to break your fast in the morning than with a super green. Kale is a great source of fiber, protein, and vitamins A, B, C, and K. This easy-to-make salad is a sure way to add an energizing boost to your morning.

// TO MAKE THE DRESSING In a small bowl, whisk together all the dressing ingredients until well blended.

// TO MAKE THE SALAD Put the kale in a large bowl and pour over the dressing. Using clean hands, massage the dressing into the kale to soften the leaves.

// Top the kale with the citrus sections, pomegranate arils, and pumpkin seeds.

TIP

Experiment with different fruits and seeds for dozens of other healthy topping options.

DRESSING

1 tablespoon Dijon mustard

Dash of freshly ground black pepper

2 tablespoons balsamic vinegar

1 tablespoon fresh lime juice

1½ teaspoons pure maple syrup

SALAD

1 small bunch kale, stemmed and chopped

1 large grapefruit, peeled and separated into sections

1 large orange, peeled and separated into sections

½ cup pomegranate arils

⅓ cup raw hulled pumpkin seeds

PART TWO

—

TIER 3 RECIPES

—

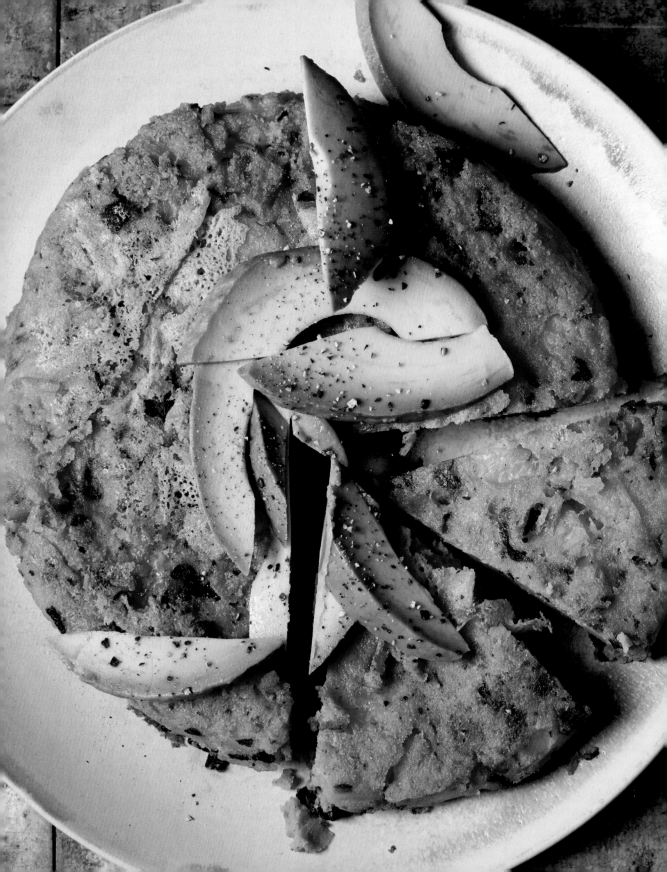

SPINACH TORTILLA (SPINACH OMELET)

SERVES
2

Spanish potato and onion omelets, known as *tortillas*, are quite common in Cuban households, and I grew up on them. This Spinach Tortilla is my healthy take on a traditional *tortilla*, minus the cholesterol and increased risk of disease that usually come from egg consumption. It's not only a great breakfast dish, but can be enjoyed for lunch or dinner, too.

2 tablespoons olive oil

⅓ small onion, minced

2 small Yukon Gold potatoes, cubed

½ cup chopped spinach

½ cup chickpea flour

¼ teaspoon sea salt, or to taste

Freshly ground black pepper

1 Hass avocado, sliced, for garnish

// In an 8-inch skillet, heat 1 tablespoon of the olive oil over medium heat. Add the onion and potato and cook for a few minutes, until vegetables are soft.

// Add the spinach and ¼ cup water and stir. Reduce the heat to medium-low, cover, and cook for 10 to 15 minutes, until the potatoes are soft.

// Meanwhile, in a medium bowl, whisk together the chickpea flour and ½ cup water. Season with the salt and pepper.

// Add the potato mixture to the chickpea flour mixture and stir to combine.

// Wipe out the skillet. Heat the remaining 1 tablespoon olive oil over medium heat. Transfer the potato–chickpea flour mixture to the pan, cover, and cook for about 5 minutes, or until golden brown on the bottom.

// Uncover the pan and set a plate larger than the diameter of the pan over the top. Holding the plate and the pan together, flip them so the tortilla falls out onto the plate. Slide the tortilla back into the pan and cook on the second side for 5 minutes. Transfer the tortilla to a serving plate.

// Top with the avocado, season with pepper, and serve.

ALMOND BUTTER AND BLUEBERRY SWEET POTATO TOAST

SERVES

2

This is a craveable, nutrient-dense breakfast. Sweet potatoes contain vitamins B_6, C, and D and are full of potassium, magnesium, and carotenoids (which boost immunity to disease and help ward off cancer). This powerhouse meal hits an even higher nutritional level when topped with blueberries and almond butter.

1 sweet potato, cut into ¼-inch-thick slices

¼ cup almond butter

½ cup blueberries

// Preheat the oven to 350°F.

// Arrange the sweet potato slices on a baking sheet. Bake until the slices are tender, about 20 minutes. (You can also cook these in a toaster, but you may need to run the toaster on high for three or four cycles.)

// Serve warm, topped with the almond butter and blueberries. Store any leftover sweet potato slices, without toppings, in an airtight container in the refrigerator for up to 1 week. Reheat in the toaster or toaster oven and top as directed.

PART
TWO

—

TIER 3
RECIPES

—

PAGE
246

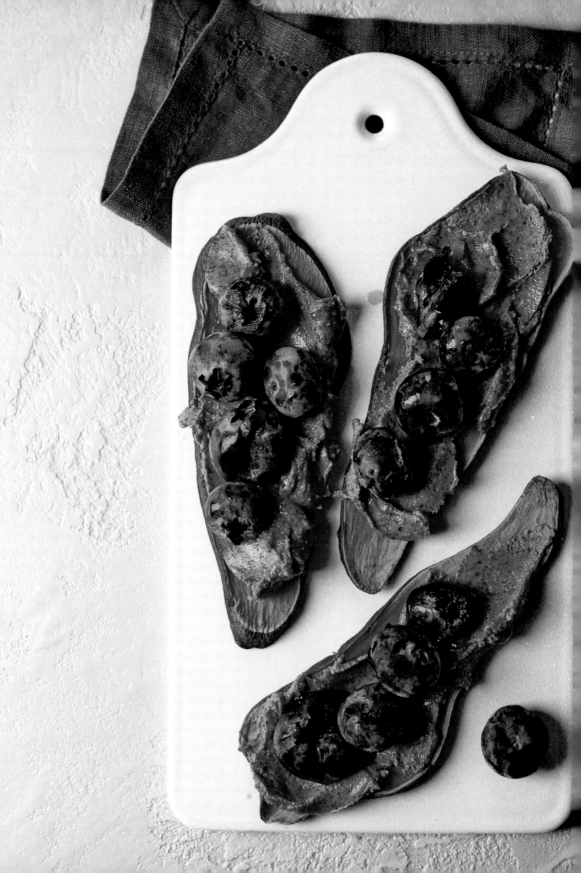

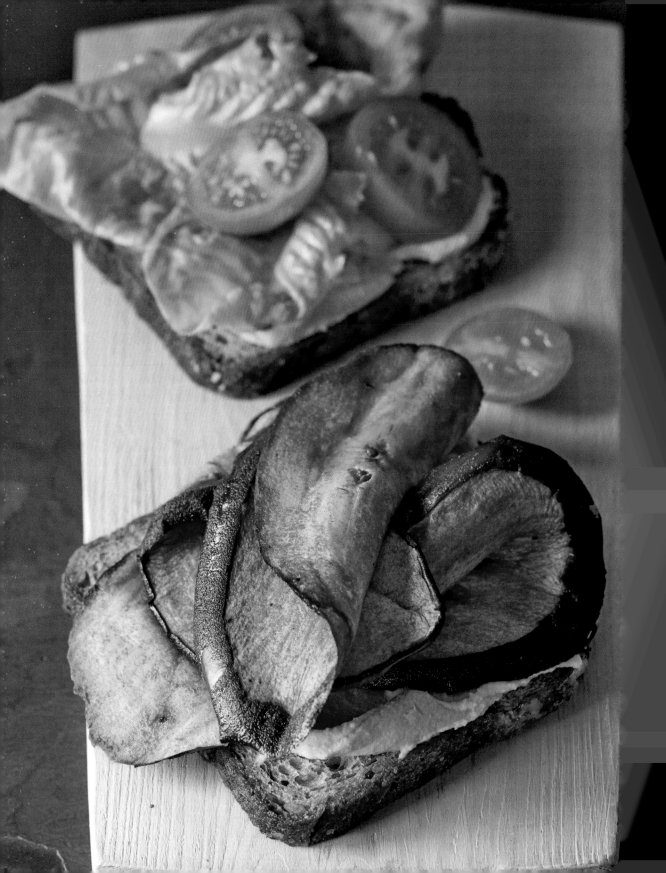

BLT BREAKFAST SANDWICH

SERVES
1

Breakfast sandwiches are quick to make and easy to eat, and this one is no exception. The crispy and meaty-tasting eggplant, juicy tomato, and crunchy bread make for a perfect pairing of flavors and textures.

// TO MAKE THE EGGPLANT "BACON" Preheat the oven to 225°F.

// In a medium bowl, whisk together the coconut aminos, maple syrup, paprika, liquid smoke, cayenne, lime juice, and black pepper.

// Arrange the eggplant slices in a single layer on a baking sheet. Brush or spoon the coconut amino mixture over both sides of each slice. Bake for 25 to 30 minutes, until slightly crispy (they will get crispier as they cool). Remove from the oven and let cool.

// TO ASSEMBLE THE SANDWICH Spread the hummus over one side of each slice of toast. Top one piece of toast with a few slices of the eggplant "bacon," the tomato, and the lettuce. Set the second piece of toast on top. Store any leftover eggplant slices in an airtight container in the refrigerator for up to 5 days.

EGGPLANT "BACON"

2 tablespoons coconut aminos

1 tablespoon pure maple syrup

1 teaspoon smoked paprika

1 teaspoon liquid smoke

¼ teaspoon cayenne pepper

2 tablespoons fresh lime juice

1 teaspoon freshly ground black pepper

1 medium eggplant, cut lengthwise into ⅛-inch-thick slices

SANDWICH

1 tablespoon hummus, store-bought or homemade (page 284)

2 slices gluten-free vegan bread, toasted

1 tomato, sliced

2 butter lettuce leaves

TIP

I've used hummus in place of traditional mayonnaise, but feel free to get creative and experiment with vegan mayo or even nondairy cheese spreads.

SWEET POTATO AND BLACK BEAN SALAD BOWL

SERVES
2

Bowls are always a great idea, and so easy to put together. This one is made with roasted sweet potato, black beans, corn, spinach, a tomato and avocado salad, and a nice scoop of hummus. This bowl can be enjoyed as is or topped with your favorite dressing.

// Preheat the oven to 400°F. Line a baking sheet with parchment paper.

// Spread the sweet potato over the prepared baking sheet. Sprinkle with the paprika and roast for about 30 minutes, flipping once halfway through, or until tender and golden.

// Meanwhile, in a medium bowl, combine the avocado, tomato, onion, lime juice, and parsley. Season with salt to taste.

// Divide the sweet potato, tomato-avocado salad, spinach, corn, and black beans between two bowls. Top with the hummus and serve.

2 small sweet potatoes, cut into 1-inch cubes

¼ teaspoon paprika

½ Hass avocado, sliced

1 large tomato, sliced

⅓ onion, diced

Juice of ½ lime

Pinch of dried parsley flakes

Sea salt

2 cups spinach

1 cup canned corn, drained and rinsed

1 cup canned black beans, drained and rinsed

¼ cup hummus, store-bought or homemade (page 284)

PART
TWO

—

TIER 3
RECIPES

—

PAGE
250

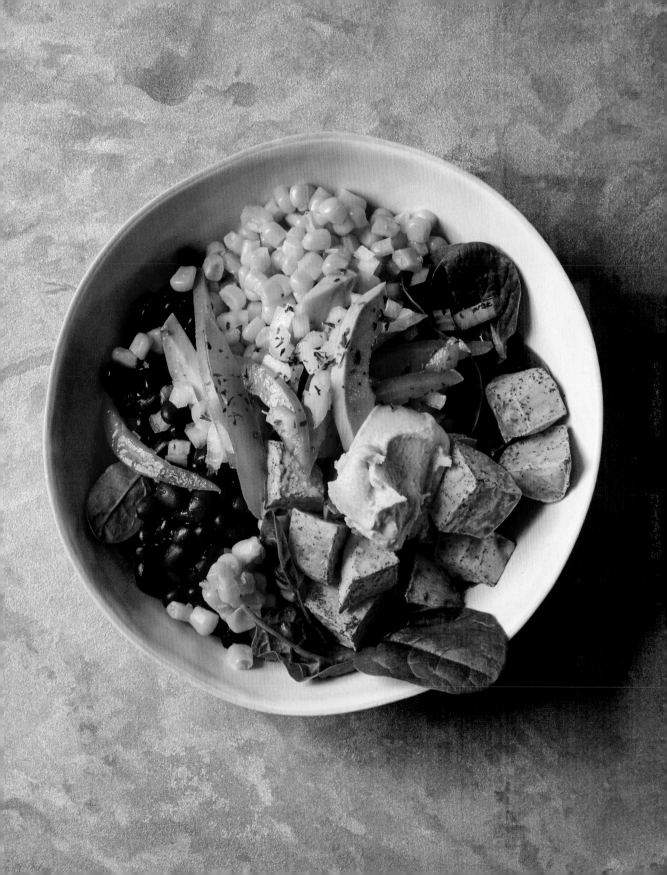

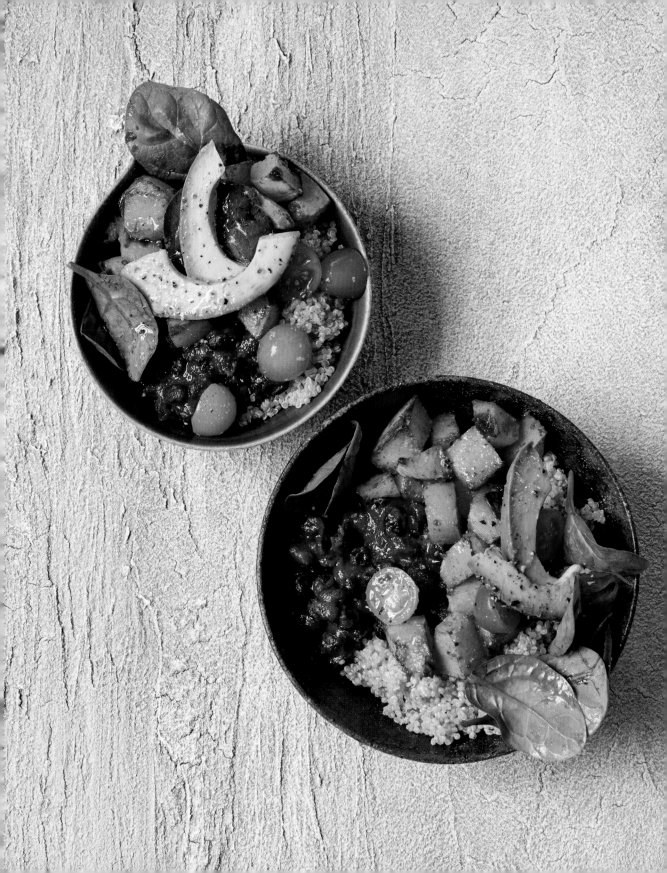

BLACK BEAN AND SQUASH QUINOA BOWL

SERVES
2

This delicious and nutritious bowl is made with butternut squash, quinoa, black beans, avocado, tomato, and spinach—all heart-healthy plant foods.

// Preheat the oven to 400°F. Line a baking sheet with parchment paper.

// Spread the butternut squash over the prepared baking sheet and sprinkle with the paprika and a pinch of salt. Roast for 30 to 35 minutes, flipping halfway through, until tender and golden brown.

// Meanwhile, rinse the quinoa in a fine-mesh sieve and drain well. Transfer the quinoa to a small saucepan and add 1 cup water and a pinch of salt. Bring to a boil, then reduce the heat to medium-low, cover with the lid slightly ajar, and simmer for 12 to 15 minutes, until the water has been absorbed. Remove from the heat, cover completely, and let stand for 5 minutes. Fluff the quinoa with a fork.

// In a separate small saucepan, stir together the black beans (with the liquid from the can), tomato paste, and a pinch of salt. Bring to a simmer over low heat and cook for about 10 minutes.

// **TO MAKE THE DRESSING** In a small bowl, whisk together the lime juice, vinegar, olive oil, and garlic powder and season with salt and pepper.

// **TO ASSEMBLE THE BOWLS** Divide the butternut squash, quinoa, black beans, spinach, tomatoes, and avocado between two bowls. Top with the dressing and serve.

2 cups cubed peeled butternut squash

½ teaspoon paprika

Sea salt

½ cup uncooked quinoa

1 cup canned black beans (do not drain)

1 tablespoon tomato paste

DRESSING

Juice of 1 lime

1½ tablespoons red wine vinegar

1 tablespoon extra-virgin olive oil

Pinch of garlic powder

Sea salt and freshly ground black pepper

BOWLS

2 cups spinach

1 cup cherry tomatoes, halved

½ avocado, sliced

TERIYAKI SUSHI BOWL

SERVES 2

All these ingredients are delicious on their own. But together, they form a bowl of awesomeness! Rich in vitamins, minerals, fiber, and flavor, this dish will quickly become a go-to staple in your home.

// Preheat the oven to 400°F. Line a baking sheet with parchment paper.

// Spread the sweet potatoes over the prepared baking sheet and roast for about 30 minutes, flipping once halfway through, until tender and golden.

// Meanwhile, in a small saucepan, combine the rice, a pinch of salt, and 1 cup water and bring to a boil. Reduce the heat to low, cover, and simmer for about 30 minutes, until the water has been absorbed. Remove from the heat and let stand, covered, for 5 to 10 minutes. Fluff the rice with a fork and set aside.

// **TO PREPARE THE TERIYAKI DRESSING** In a small bowl, whisk together the teriyaki sauce, mayo, and coconut aminos.

// **TO ASSEMBLE THE BOWLS** Divide the sweet potato, rice, carrots, radishes, avocado, and kale between two bowls. Top with the scallions, pickled ginger, dulse flakes, and sesame seeds. Drizzle with the dressing and serve.

2 sweet potatoes, peeled and cut into 1-inch cubes (about 2 cups)

½ cup uncooked sprouted short-grain brown rice

Sea salt

TERIYAKI DRESSING

2½ tablespoons coconut amino-based teriyaki sauce

1 tablespoon vegan soy-free mayo

2 teaspoons coconut aminos

BOWLS

2 carrots, shredded or thinly sliced

2 radishes, sliced

1 Hass avocado, sliced

2 cups chopped stemmed kale leaves or other greens

2 scallions, sliced

Pickled ginger

Dulse flakes

Sesame seeds

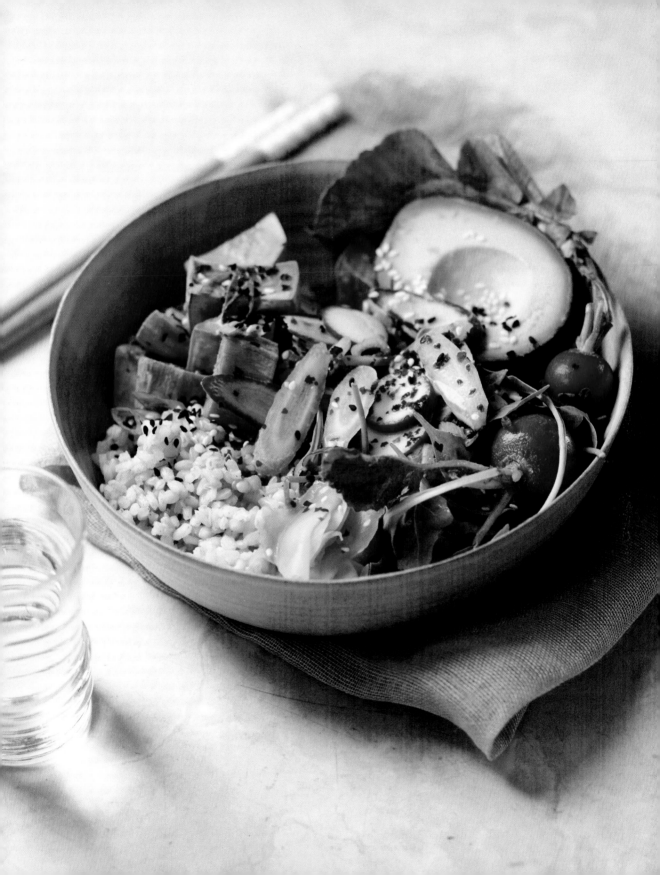

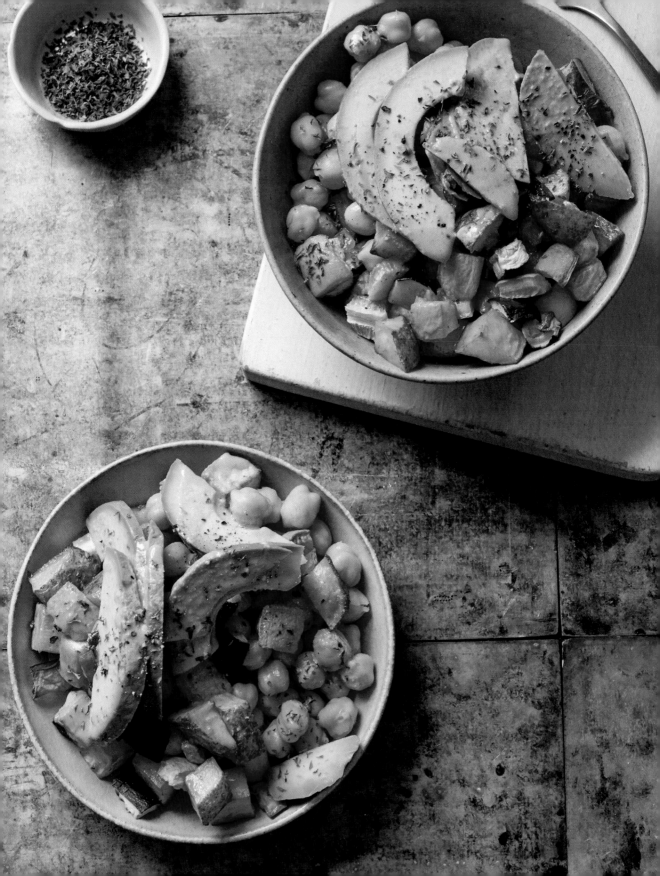

ZUCCHINI AND SQUASH POTATO BOWL

SERVES
2

Here's a powerhouse of foods in one bowl. Chickpeas are a great source of protein, fiber, magnesium, potassium, folate, and fiber. Squash and zucchini are loaded with inflammation-fighting vitamins and minerals. Put them together with luscious Yukon Gold potatoes, and you've got a filling, high-flavor dish that's great for lunch or dinner.

// Preheat the oven to 400°F. Line a large baking sheet with parchment paper.

// In a medium bowl, toss together the potatoes, canola oil, coconut aminos, cumin, and a pinch of salt. Spread the potatoes over the prepared baking sheet and roast for 15 minutes. Remove the baking sheet from the oven, flip the potatoes, and push them aside to make enough room for the squash and zucchini. Put the squash and zucchini on the baking sheet, season with a pinch of sea salt, and return the baking sheet to the oven. Roast for 15 to 20 minutes, until the potatoes are tender.

// **MEANWHILE, TO MAKE THE DRESSING** In a small bowl, whisk together the tahini, lemon juice, vinegar, coconut aminos, garlic powder, and pepper. Season with salt.

// **TO ASSEMBLE THE BOWLS** Divide the potatoes, squash, zucchini, chickpeas, and avocado between two bowls. Top with the parsley and season with pepper. Drizzle with the dressing and serve.

2 medium Yukon Gold potatoes (about 10 ounces), cubed

1 tablespoon canola oil

1 tablespoon coconut aminos

Pinch of ground cumin

Sea salt

1 yellow squash, cubed

1 zucchini, cubed

TAHINI DRESSING

1 tablespoon tahini

Juice of 1 lemon

1 tablespoon balsamic vinegar

1 teaspoon coconut aminos

¼ teaspoon garlic powder

Pinch of freshly ground black pepper

Sea salt

BOWLS

1 (15-ounce) can chickpeas, drained and rinsed

1 Hass avocado, sliced

Parsley flakes

Freshly ground black pepper

PART
TWO

—

TIER 3
RECIPES

—

RAINBOW QUINOA BOWL

SERVES

2

This colorful and nutritious quinoa bowl is loaded with protein, vitamins, and fiber! There's no better way to eat your veggies. The quinoa, kale, chickpeas, corn, tomato, and avocado pair perfectly for a meal that is complete, balanced, and full of flavor.

// Rinse the quinoa in a fine-mesh colander and drain well. Transfer the quinoa to a small saucepan and add 1⅓ cups water and a pinch of salt. Bring to a boil, then reduce the heat to medium-low, cover, and simmer for 12 to 15 minutes, until the water has been absorbed. Remove from the heat, and let stand, covered, for 5 minutes. Uncover and fluff the quinoa with a fork.

// **TO MAKE THE DRESSING** In a small bowl, whisk together the tahini, lemon juice, garlic powder, salt, and 2 tablespoons water.

// **TO ASSEMBLE THE BOWLS** Divide the quinoa, kale, carrots, tomatoes, avocado, chickpeas, and corn between two bowls. Season with salt and pepper. Top with the dressing, garnish with sesame seeds, and serve.

⅔ **cup uncooked quinoa**

Sea salt

LEMON-TAHINI DRESSING

1½ **tablespoons tahini**

Juice of ½ lemon

Pinch of garlic powder

¼ **teaspoon sea salt**

BOWLS

2 **cups chopped stemmed kale leaves**

2 **carrots, shredded (about 1 cup)**

1 **cup cherry tomatoes, halved**

½ **Hass avocado, sliced**

1 **cup canned chickpeas, drained and rinsed**

1 **cup canned sweet corn, drained and rinsed**

Sea salt and freshly ground black pepper

Sesame seeds

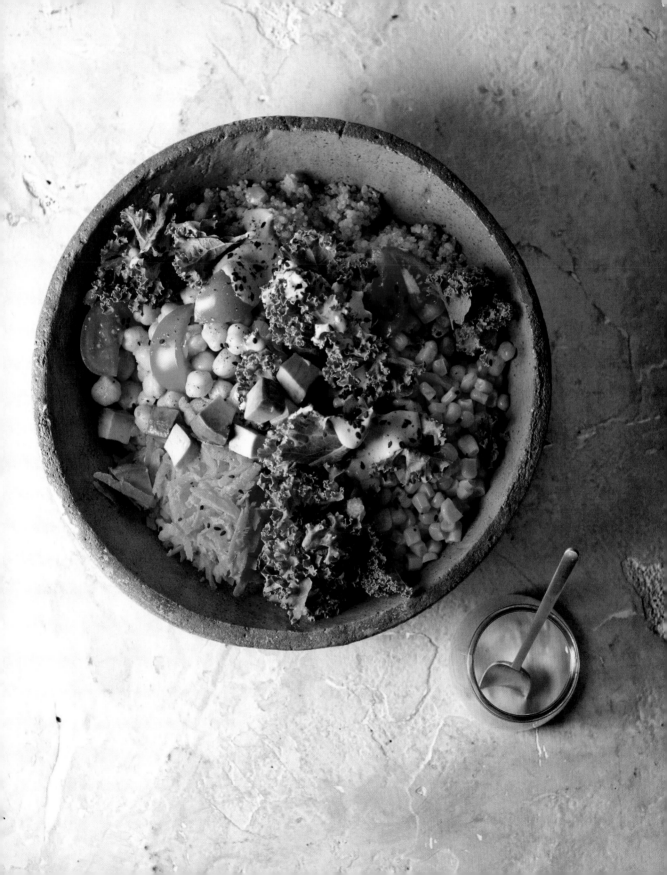

GRILLED ARTICHOKE AND BLACK BEAN BOWL

SERVES

2

The smoky flavor of the grilled artichokes and the tanginess of the salsa pair deliciously with the black beans and quinoa. This recipe uses jarred grilled artichokes, but if you're not pressed for time, feel free to cook fresh ones and use those instead.

// Rinse the quinoa in a fine-mesh sieve and drain well. Transfer the quinoa to a small saucepan and add 1 cup water and a pinch of salt. Bring to a boil, then reduce the heat to medium-low, cover, and simmer for 12 to 15 minutes, until the water has been absorbed. Remove from the heat and let stand, covered, for 5 minutes. Uncover and fluff the quinoa with a fork.

// Meanwhile, in a small saucepan, combine the black beans (with the reserved liquid from the can), tomato paste, onion powder, garlic powder, and a pinch of salt. Bring to a simmer over low heat and cook for about 10 minutes, until heated through.

// **TO MAKE THE SALSA** In a small bowl, combine the bell pepper, tomato, and onion. Add the vinegar, lime juice, and paprika and season with salt and black pepper. Toss to combine.

// Divide the quinoa, black beans, and artichokes between two bowls. Top with the salsa and serve!

½ cup uncooked quinoa

Sea salt

2 cups canned black beans, drained (liquid reserved) and rinsed

1 tablespoon tomato paste

Pinch of onion powder

Pinch of garlic powder

FOR SALSA

1 bell pepper, diced

1 tomato, chopped

½ onion, diced

2 tablespoons distilled white vinegar

Juice of ½ lime

¼ teaspoon paprika

Sea salt and freshly ground black pepper

4 jarred marinated grilled artichokes, drained

PART
TWO

—

TIER 3
RECIPES

—

PAGE

260

SUGAR SNAP PEA AND CARROT NOODLES

SERVES

2

What I love about sugar snap peas is that you don't have to shell, seed, peel, or chop them—they're enjoyed pod and all. Plus, they're loaded with vitamins, iron, and protein. This dish pairs the peas with carrots for a taste explosion, not to mention high-powered nutrition.

// TO MAKE THE DRESSING In a medium bowl, whisk together all the dressing ingredients. Set aside.

// Set a steamer basket in a large saucepan and add water to come just below the bottom of the basket. Bring the water to a simmer over medium heat. Put the broccoli in the steamer, cover, and cook for 2 minutes. Transfer the broccoli to a large bowl. Repeat to cook the carrot, then the snap peas, adding them to the bowl with the broccoli as they are done.

// Meanwhile, in a separate medium saucepan, bring 4 cups water to a boil. As soon as the water begins to boil, add the rice noodles and cook for 10 minutes, or until soft but still firm. Drain the noodles, rinse under cold running water, and drain again. Transfer the noodles to the bowl with the vegetables.

// Add the dressing and toss to combine.

// Garnish with the sesame seeds and serve. Store any leftover dressing in an airtight container in the refrigerator for up to 5 days.

DRESSING

¼ cup coconut aminos

2 tablespoons peanut butter

2 tablespoons fresh lime juice

1 teaspoon grated fresh ginger

1 tablespoon pure maple syrup

1 cup chopped broccoli

1 large carrot, shredded

2 cups sugar snap peas

8 ounces rice noodles

¼ cup sesame seeds

PART TWO

TIER 3 RECIPES

SPINACH AND KALE PASTA WITH CRISPY BRUSSELS SPROUTS

SERVES
2

This quick-and-easy pasta is tossed with a spinach-kale pesto and topped off with delicious crispy Brussels sprouts for a boost of veggie power. Truly a delicious combination that's fulfilling and flavorful!

// Preheat the oven to 450ºF. Line a baking sheet with parchment paper.

// Bring a large pot of water to a boil.

// **TO MAKE THE CRISPY BRUSSELS SPROUTS** In a small bowl, toss together the Brussels sprouts, olive oil, salt, and pepper to taste. Spread the Brussels sprouts on the prepared baking sheet and roast for 10 to 15 minutes, until crisp.

// Meanwhile, add the pasta and a pinch of salt to the boiling water and stir. Cook the pasta according to the package instructions. Drain the pasta, reserving 1/2 cup of the cooking water, and return the pasta to the pot.

// **TO PREPARE THE PESTO** In a food processor, combine the spinach, kale, 1/4 cup of the reserved pasta cooking water, the cashews, basil, olive oil, lime juice, garlic, salt, and pepper to taste. Process until smooth. If needed, add more pasta cooking water 1 tablespoon at a time until the desired consistency is reached.

// Add the pesto to the pot with the pasta and toss until the pasta is fully coated. Taste and adjust the seasoning if necessary.

// Serve the pasta topped with the crispy Brussels sprouts.

CRISPY BRUSSELS SPROUTS

1 cup shaved Brussels sprouts

1½ teaspoons olive oil

Pinch of sea salt

Freshly ground black pepper

1½ cups uncooked brown rice penne or other gluten-free vegan pasta

SPINACH AND KALE PESTO

1½ cups fresh spinach

1½ cups chopped stemmed kale leaves

2 tablespoons cashews

1 tablespoon dried basil

2 tablespoons extra-virgin olive oil

Juice of ½ lime

1 teaspoon minced garlic

¼ teaspoon sea salt

Freshly ground black pepper

PART
TWO

—

TIER 3
RECIPES

—

PAGE
262

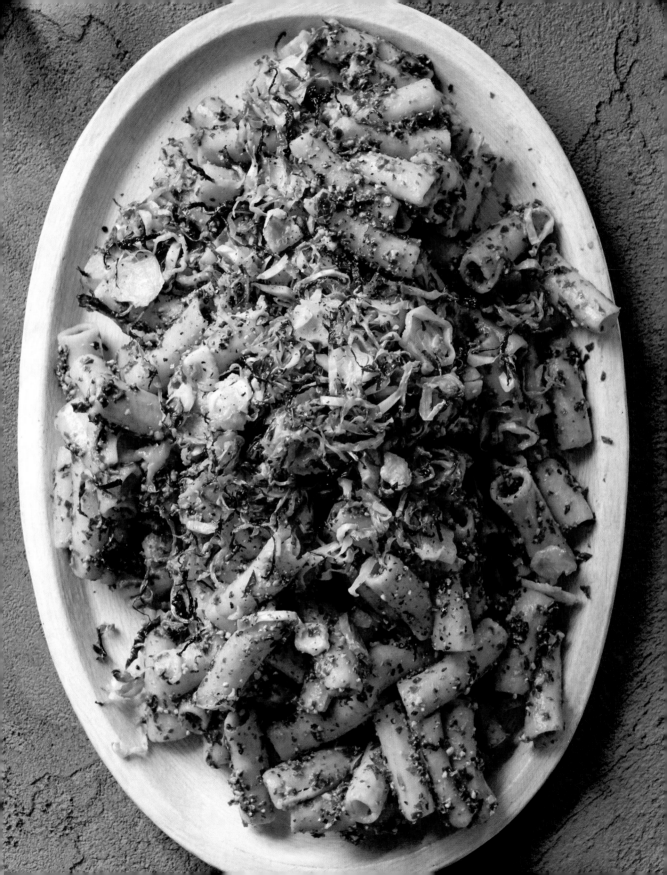

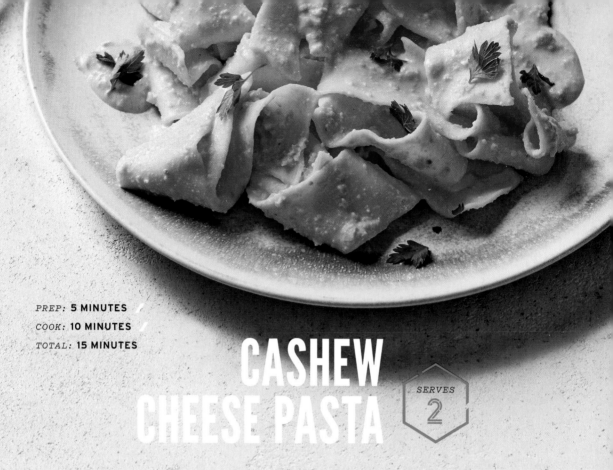

PREP: **5 MINUTES**

COOK: **10 MINUTES**

TOTAL: **15 MINUTES**

CASHEW CHEESE PASTA

SERVES
2

A simple combination of cashews, lime, and nutritional yeast makes this a healthy protein-packed meal. The cashew pieces in the sauce give the pasta a nice chunky consistency, while the fresh parsley balances and brightens the flavor.

// Put the cashews in a small bowl, add warm or hot filtered water to cover, and set aside to soak for about 5 minutes. (For a smoother consistency, soak the cashews overnight in filtered water.)

// Bring a large pot of water to a boil. Add the pasta and cook according to the package instructions.

// Meanwhile, drain the cashews and transfer them to a high-speed blender or food processor. Add the nutritional yeast, lime juice, garlic powder, salt, and $1/2$ cup water and blend until smooth.

// Drain the pasta and return it to the pot. Add the cashew sauce and toss to coat the pasta.

// Garnish with parsley, if desired, and serve.

½ cup raw cashews

2 cups uncooked gluten-free pasta

¼ cup nutritional yeast

Juice of 1 lime

Pinch of garlic powder

¼ teaspoon sea salt

Fresh parsley, for garnish (optional)

SPINACH CREAM PASTA

SERVES
2

Indulge in this easy-to-make, creamy, hearty, and delicious pasta! This kid-approved meal is made with superstar ingredients like spinach, cashews, lime juice, and nutritional yeast.

// Put the cashews in a small bowl, add warm or hot filtered water to cover, and set aside to soak for about 5 minutes. (For a smoother consistency, soak the cashews overnight in filtered water.)

// Bring a large pot of water to a boil. Add the pasta and cook according to the package instructions.

// Meanwhile, drain the cashews and transfer them to a high-speed blender or food processor. Add the spinach, nutritional yeast, lime juice, garlic powder, salt, and 1/2 cup water and blend until smooth.

// Drain the pasta and return it to the pot. Add the spinach sauce and toss to coat the pasta.

// Season with pepper and serve.

½ cup raw cashews

2 cups uncooked pasta, any shape

3 cups fresh spinach

¼ cup nutritional yeast

Juice of ½ lime

Pinch of garlic powder

¼ teaspoon sea salt

Freshly ground black pepper

PART
TWO

—

TIER 3
RECIPES

—

PAGE
265

QUINOA VEGGIE SALAD WITH SUNFLOWER SEED "PARMESAN"

SERVES
4

I love quinoa and chickpeas—especially together in the same dish. I've added pinto beans for an extra kick of protein. The sunflower seed "Parmesan" amplifies the flavors.

// Rinse the quinoa in a fine-mesh sieve and drain well. Transfer the quinoa to a small saucepan and add a pinch of salt and 2 cups water. Bring to a boil, then reduce the heat to medium-low, cover, and simmer for 12 to 15 minutes, until the water has been absorbed. Remove from the heat and let stand, covered, for 5 minutes. Uncover and fluff the quinoa with a fork and let cool.

// Put the frozen peas in a colander and set them under cool running water to thaw. Drain the peas well and transfer to a large bowl.

// Add the parsley, chickpeas, corn, pinto beans, bell peppers, celery, lime juice, and olive oil and season with salt and black pepper. Toss to combine.

// Add the cooled quinoa to the bean mixture and toss to combine.

// **TO MAKE THE SUNFLOWER SEED "PARMESAN"** In a food processor, combine all the sunflower seed "Parmesan" ingredients and pulse a few times until broken down to the consistency of grated Parmesan.

// Top the quinoa veggie salad with the "Parmesan" and serve.

1 cup uncooked quinoa

Sea salt

1 cup frozen peas

Leaves from ½ bunch parsley, minced

1 (15-ounce) can chickpeas, drained and rinsed

1 (15-ounce) can sweet corn, drained and rinsed

1 (15-ounce) pinto beans, drained and rinsed

1 green bell pepper, minced

1 red bell pepper, minced

1 small celery stalk, minced

Juice of 1 lime

2 tablespoons extra-virgin olive oil

Freshly ground black pepper

SUNFLOWER SEED "PARMESAN"

¼ cup roasted unsalted sunflower seeds

2 tablespoons nutritional yeast

¼ teaspoon sea salt

PART
TWO

—

TIER 3
RECIPES

—

ENTRÉES

—

MAIN DISH
SALADS

—

PAGE
266

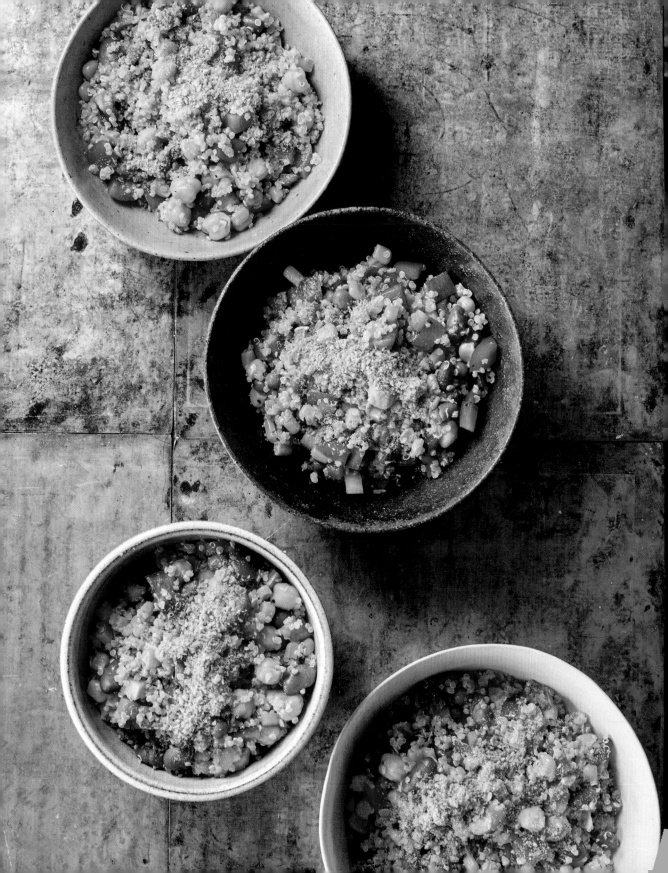

THAI PEANUT AND QUINOA SALAD

SERVES
2

This Thai-inspired crunchy salad is light, flavorful, and packed with nutritious veggies like arugula, cabbage, and carrot, all tossed with a creamy peanut dressing.

// Rinse the quinoa in a fine-mesh sieve and drain well. Transfer the quinoa to a small saucepan and add a pinch of salt and 1^1/$_3$ cups water. Bring to a boil, then reduce the heat to medium-low, cover, and simmer for 12 to 15 minutes, until the water has been absorbed. Remove from the heat and let stand, covered, for 5 minutes. Uncover and fluff the quinoa with a fork and let cool.

// **TO MAKE THE PEANUT DRESSING** In a small bowl, whisk together all the dressing ingredients until smooth.

// In a large bowl, combine the cooled quinoa, arugula, cabbage, and carrot. Add half the dressing and toss to coat the vegetables. Taste and adjust the salt if necessary.

// Top the salad with the chopped peanuts, drizzle with the remaining dressing, and serve.

^{2}/$_3$ cup uncooked quinoa

Sea salt

PEANUT DRESSING

2 tablespoons peanut butter

1 tablespoon coconut aminos

2 tablespoons rice vinegar

Pinch of ground ginger

Pinch of freshly ground black pepper

2 cups arugula

½ cup shredded cabbage

1 carrot, shredded

2 tablespoons chopped raw peanuts

PART
TWO

—

TIER 3
RECIPES

—

ENTRÉES

—

MAIN DISH
SALADS

—

PAGE
268

THE FUTURE DEPENDS ON WHAT WE DO IN THE PRESENT.

—MAHATMA GANDHI

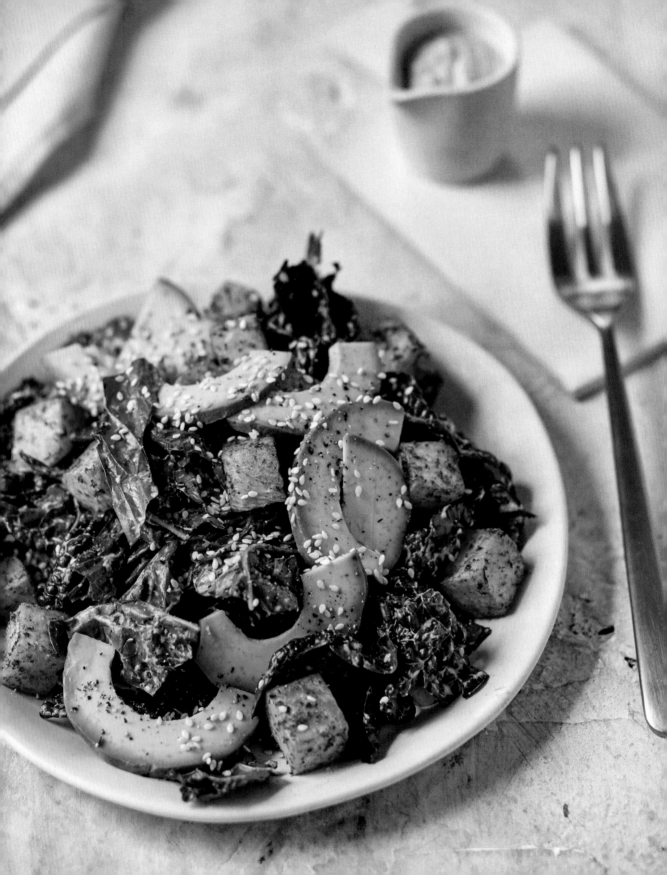

ROASTED RUTABAGA AND KALE SALAD

SERVES
2

Rutabaga is a nutrient-rich vegetable that's high in antioxidant compounds. Here it's seasoned with herbs and spices served over a kale salad, dressed in a creamy cashew dressing, and topped with sesame seeds. If you can't find rutabaga in your local store (or if they're not in season), feel free to sub in sweet potatoes, which are available all year long in many places.

// Preheat the oven to 425°F. Line a baking sheet with parchment paper.

// Put the cashews in a small bowl, add warm or hot filtered water to cover, and set aside to soak for 2 to 3 hours.

// In a medium bowl, toss together the rutabagas, olive oil, paprika, cumin, coriander, garlic powder, basil, and parsley and season with salt. Spread the rutabagas over the prepared baking sheet and roast for 35 to 40 minutes, until fork-tender and golden.

// **TO MAKE THE DRESSING** Drain and rinse the cashews and transfer them to a high-speed blender or food processor. Add the nutritional yeast, lemon juice, mustard, salt, garlic powder, and 2 tablespoons water. Blend until creamy and smooth.

// Put the kale in a large bowl and add the dressing. Using clean hands, massage the dressing into the kale until fully coated.

// Top the kale with the rutabaga, avocado, and sesame seeds and serve.

¼ cup raw cashews

2 small rutabagas, peeled and cut into 1-inch pieces (about 2 cups)

1 tablespoon olive oil

¼ teaspoon smoked paprika

¼ teaspoon ground cumin

¼ teaspoon ground coriander

¼ teaspoon garlic powder

¼ teaspoon dried basil

½ teaspoon dried parsley flakes

Sea salt

DRESSING

2 teaspoons nutritional yeast

Juice of ½ lemon

½ teaspoon Dijon mustard

¼ teaspoon sea salt

Pinch of garlic powder

4 cups chopped stemmed kale leaves

1 Hass avocado, sliced

Sesame seeds

PART
TWO

—

TIER 3
RECIPES

—

ENTRÉES

—

MAIN DISH
SALADS

ENTRÉES
OTHER

LENTIL AND BEAN CHILI SOUP

SERVES
4

Lentils are packed with an array of nutrients that support health and metabolism. In this recipe, I've turned them into a chili soup that is out of this world. We love keeping fresh batches of it in our fridge and hope you enjoy it as much as we do.

// In a large pot, combine the lentils, kidney beans, onion, garlic, cumin, and coriander. Add 8 cups water. Bring to a boil, reduce the heat to medium-low, cover, and simmer, stirring occasionally, for about 45 minutes.

// Add the corn, bell peppers, tomato, tomato paste, chili powder, salt, and black pepper, stir, and cook for 30 minutes, or longer for a thicker chili. Taste and adjust the seasoning, and add water if necessary to thin the chili to the desired consistency.

// Ladle the chili into bowls and top each with a few slices of avocado. Garnish with cilantro, if desired, and serve.

1 cup dry lentils, rinsed

1 cup dry red kidney beans or pinto beans, rinsed

½ small white onion, finely chopped

1 garlic clove, minced

1 tablespoon ground cumin

1 tablespoon ground coriander

1 (15-ounce) can sweet corn, drained and rinsed

½ small green bell pepper, minced

½ small red bell pepper, minced

1 tomato, chopped

2 tablespoons tomato paste

1 teaspoon chili powder

¾ teaspoon sea salt, or to taste

½ teaspoon freshly ground black pepper

1 Hass avocado, sliced, for serving

Fresh cilantro, for garnish (optional)

PART
TWO

—

TIER 3
RECIPES

—

ENTRÉES

—

OTHER

—

PAGE
272

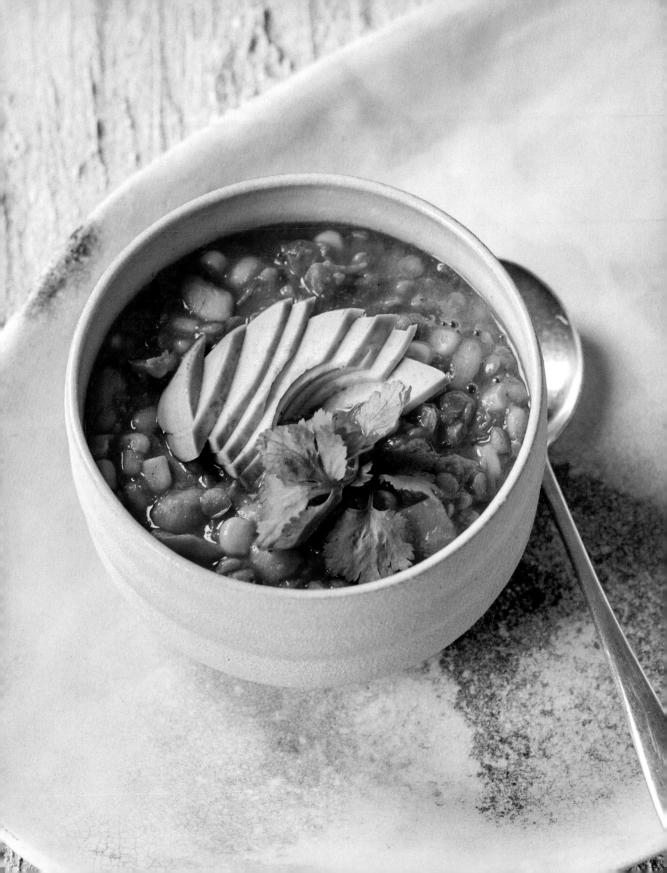

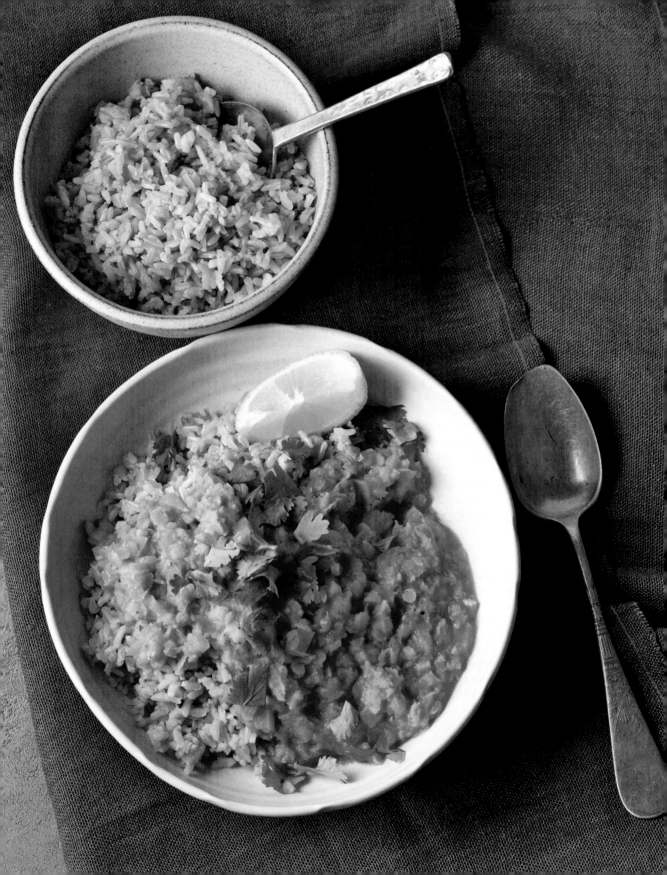

RED LENTIL DAL

SERVES
4

Dal is a classic lentil-based Indian dish that is simple to prepare and wonderful to enjoy. Serve it often, and it is destined to become a family favorite.

// In a medium-large pot, combine the lentils, bell pepper, onion, garlic, ginger, lemon juice, curry powder, cumin, black pepper, turmeric, and 3 cups water. Bring to a boil. Reduce the heat to low, cover, and simmer, stirring occasionally, for 30 minutes, or until the lentils are soft.

// Spoon the rice or quinoa into a serving bowl or platter and top with the dal. Garnish with cilantro, if desired, and serve with lemon wedges (for squeezing).

1 cup dry red lentils

1 yellow bell pepper, chopped

1 small red onion, chopped

1 tablespoon minced garlic

1 teaspoon minced fresh ginger

Juice of 1 lemon

1 teaspoon curry powder

1 tablespoon ground cumin

¼ teaspoon freshly ground black pepper

1 teaspoon ground turmeric

Cooked brown rice or quinoa, for serving

Fresh cilantro, for garnish (optional)

Lemon wedges

PART TWO

—

TIER 3 RECIPES

—

ENTRÉES

—

OTHER

—

PAGE
275

SAUTÉED BELUGA LENTILS AND BUTTERNUT SQUASH

SERVES
2

Beluga lentils are black, tiny, and round and hold their shape well when cooked (unlike other lentils, which can become mushy). I love to sauté them and pair them with roasted butternut squash, because of its sweet, nutty taste. Try whipping up a larger batch for leftovers during the week.

// TO MAKE THE BUTTERNUT SQUASH Preheat the oven to 425°F. Line a baking sheet with parchment paper.

// In a large bowl, toss together the squash, olive oil, oregano, curry powder, and salt and pepper to taste, until the squash is evenly coated. Spread the squash in a single layer over the prepared baking sheet. Roast for 30 to 35 minutes, until tender and golden brown, flipping once halfway through the cooking time. Remove from the oven and set aside.

// TO MAKE THE LENTILS In a small saucepan, bring 1$1/2$ cups water to a boil. Add the lentils and a pinch of salt, reduce the heat to maintain a simmer, and cook, uncovered, for 25 to 30 minutes, until tender. Drain in a colander. Rinse and drain.

// In the same saucepan, heat the olive oil over medium heat. Add the garlic and cook until the garlic is lightly crisp. Add the lentils and cook, stirring occasionally, for about 5 minutes, or until warmed through. Transfer the lentils to a medium bowl.

// Add the red onion, vinegar, lime juice, mustard, basil, and parsley and toss to combine. Add the roasted squash and the arugula and toss again.

// Transfer to a serving dish and serve.

BUTTERNUT SQUASH

3 cups cubed peeled butternut squash

1 tablespoon olive oil

2 teaspoons dried oregano

1 teaspoon curry powder

Sea salt and freshly ground black pepper

LENTILS

¾ cup dry black beluga lentils, rinsed

Sea salt

1 tablespoon olive oil

1 tablespoon minced garlic

½ small red onion, diced

1 tablespoon cider vinegar

Juice of ½ lime

1 teaspoon Dijon mustard

1½ tablespoons dried basil

1 tablespoon parsley flakes

1 cup arugula or other greens

PART TWO

———

TIER 3 RECIPES

———

ENTRÉES

———

OTHER

———

PAGE

276

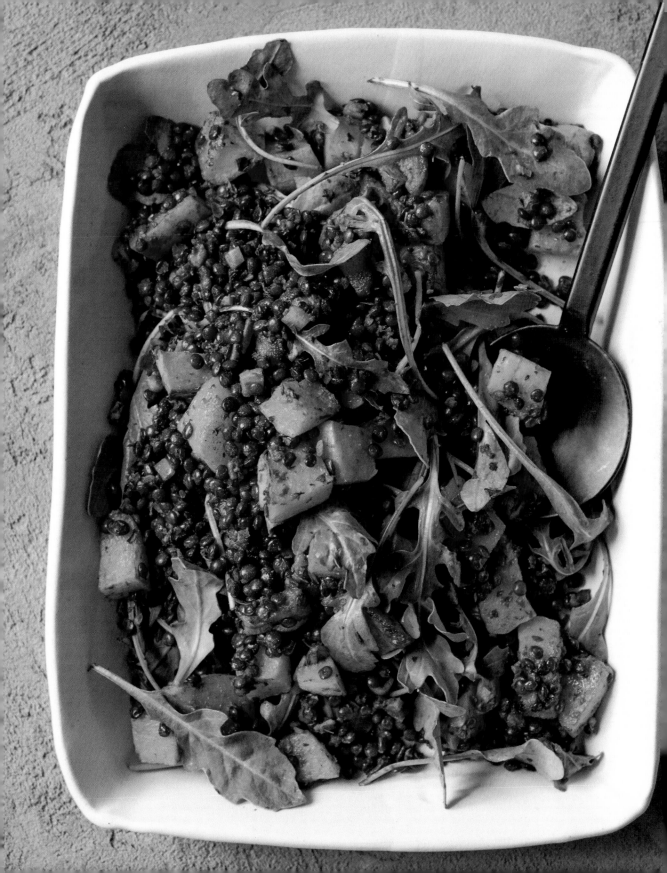

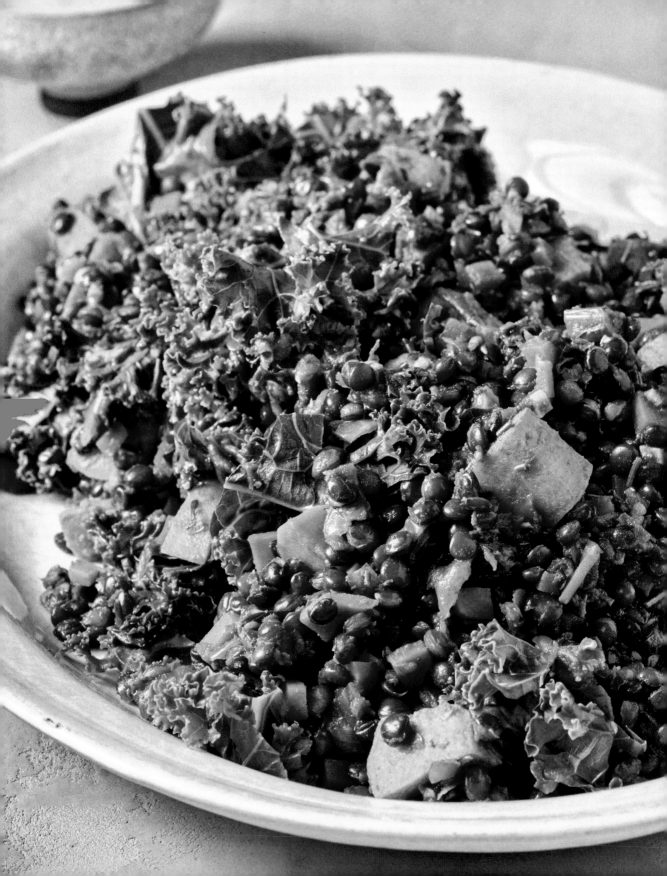

BRAISED BELUGA LENTILS WITH KALE

SERVES

2

1 tablespoon extra-virgin olive oil

1 carrot, diced

1 celery stalk, diced

1 yellow onion, diced

2 garlic cloves, minced

1 cup dry black beluga lentils

1 tablespoon dried rosemary

1 teaspoon ground coriander

1 teaspoon ground cumin

⅛ teaspoon ground turmeric

⅛ teaspoon ground ginger

2 cups vegetable broth

2 large ripe tomatoes, chopped

1 (8-ounce) sweet potato, peeled and cut into 1-inch cubes (about 1 cup)

½ bunch kale, stemmed and coarsely chopped (about 2 cups)

1 tablespoon sherry vinegar

¼ teaspoon sea salt, plus more as needed

Pinch of freshly ground black pepper, or to taste

½ cup plain coconut milk yogurt or other nondairy yogurt

Juice of ¼ lemon

This rosemary-infused braised lentil recipe is definitely a crowd-pleaser. The beluga lentils are simmered in a tomato-and-vegetable-based broth, making this dish hearty and flavorful!

// In a medium pot, heat the olive oil over medium heat. Add the carrot, celery, onion, and garlic. Cook, stirring occasionally, for a few minutes, until softened and fragrant.

// Stir in the lentils, rosemary, coriander, cumin, turmeric, and ginger and cook for 1 to 2 minutes.

// Add the broth, tomatoes, and sweet potato. Bring to a boil. Reduce the heat to medium-low and simmer for 25 to 30 minutes, until the lentils are tender. If necessary, add water, ½ cup at a time, until the desired consistency is reached. Taste and adjust the seasoning.

// Stir in the kale and vinegar and simmer for a few minutes more, until the kale has wilted.

// In a small bowl, stir together the yogurt, lemon juice, sea salt, and pepper.

// Serve the lentils topped with the yogurt sauce.

PART TWO

———

TIER 3 RECIPES

———

ENTRÉES

———

OTHER

———

SPICY BBQ GRILLED EGGPLANT STEAKS

SERVES
2

If you've had difficulty finding an eggplant recipe you love, your search is over. This is an easy dish to make and is as satisfying as it is nutritious. The BBQ sauce adds a touch of tang that leaves you wanting more.

// In a small saucepan, combine the rice, a pinch of salt, and 1⅓ cups water. Bring to a boil. Reduce the heat to low, cover, and simmer for about 20 minutes. Remove from the heat and let stand, covered, for 5 minutes more.

// TO MAKE THE EGGPLANT In a small bowl, whisk together the coconut aminos, olive oil, lime juice, coriander, cumin, paprika, thyme, cayenne, black pepper, salt, scallion, and garlic.

// Brush both sides of each eggplant slice with the coconut amino mixture.

// Lightly grease a grill pan with olive oil and heat it over medium-high heat. Working in batches, add the eggplant and cook for 3 to 5 minutes on each side, until golden brown.

⅔ cup uncooked jasmine rice

Sea salt

EGGPLANT

2 tablespoons coconut aminos

1 tablespoon extra-virgin olive oil, plus more as needed

Juice of 1 lime

1 tablespoon ground coriander

2 teaspoons ground cumin

1 teaspoon smoked paprika

1 teaspoon dried thyme

Pinch of cayenne pepper

Pinch of freshly ground black pepper, or to taste

Pinch of sea salt, or to taste

1 scallion, thinly sliced

1 garlic clove, minced, or ¼ teaspoon garlic powder

1 large or 2 small eggplants, sliced lengthwise into ½-inch-thick "steaks"

PART TWO

—

TIER 3 RECIPES

—

ENTRÉES

—

OTHER

—

PAGE
280

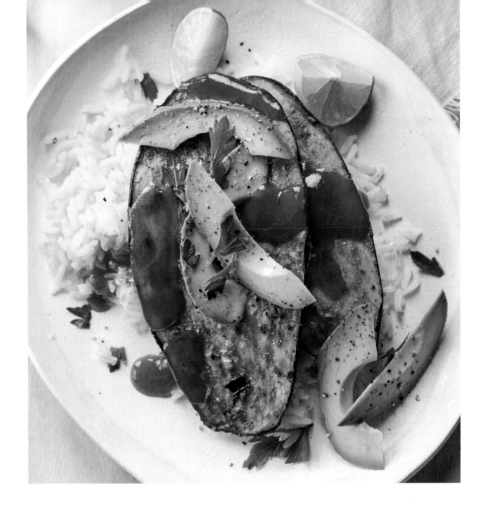

BBQ SAUCE

2 tablespoons store-bought vegan barbecue sauce

1 teaspoon liquid smoke

Juice of ½ lime

Pinch of sea salt, or to taste

Pinch of freshly ground black pepper, or to taste

TO SERVE

½ avocado, sliced (optional)

Lime wedges, for garnish

Fresh parsley, for garnish

// **MEANWHILE, TO MAKE THE BBQ SAUCE** In a small bowl, whisk together the barbecue sauce, liquid smoke, lime juice, salt, and pepper. Taste and adjust the seasoning if necessary.

// Scoop the rice onto two plates and top with the grilled eggplant steaks and the avocado, if desired. Garnish with lime wedges and parsley and serve with the BBQ sauce on the side. Store any leftovers in an airtight container in the refrigerator for up to 3 days.

BLACK BEANS AND YUCA WITH JASMINE RICE AND AVOCADO

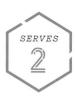

SERVES

2

This delicious meal is Latin-inspired, using culture favorites such as avocado (*aguacate*), black beans (*frijoles negros*), cassava (yuca), and rice (*arroz*). It's the perfect blend of heart-healthy carbohydrates, protein, fiber, vitamins, and minerals and makes for a complete meal any time of day.

// In a medium saucepan, combine the refried black beans, cassava, cumin, lime juice, a pinch of salt, and 2 cups water. Bring to a boil, then reduce the heat to maintain a simmer. Cook, breaking up the cassava into smaller pieces with a spoon, for about 25 minutes, or until the cassava is tender.

// In a separate small saucepan, combine the rice, a pinch of salt, and 1 1/3 cups water and bring to a boil. Reduce the heat to low, cover, and simmer for about 20 minutes. Remove from the heat and let stand, covered, for 5 minutes. Fluff the rice with a fork.

// Serve the bean mixture over the rice. Garnish with sliced avocado, cilantro, or parsley, if desired, and serve.

1½ cups canned vegetarian refried black beans

2 pieces frozen cassava (yuca)

1 tablespoon ground cumin

Juice of ½ lime

Sea salt

⅔ cup uncooked jasmine rice

½ avocado, sliced

Fresh cilantro or parsley, for garnish (optional)

PART TWO

—

TIER 3 RECIPES

—

ENTRÉES

—

OTHER

—

PAGE

282

VEGGIE FRIED RICE

SERVES

2

Enjoy this nutritious veggie-loaded rice as is or with a side of sliced avocado. Its delicious and creamy texture complements any dish. We can never get enough of it in our home.

// In a small saucepan, combine the rice, a pinch of salt, and 2 cups water. Bring to a boil. Reduce the heat to low, cover, and simmer for about 30 minutes. Remove from the heat and let stand, covered, for 5 to 10 minutes. Fluff the rice with a fork and set aside.

// In a large skillet, heat the sesame oil over medium heat. Add the garlic and ginger and cook, stirring continuously, for 1 minute.

// Add the carrots, peas, corn, broccoli, scallion, coconut aminos, and vinegar and cook, stirring frequently, for a few minutes more.

// Add the rice and a pinch of salt and cook until well combined and warmed through.

// Garnish with sesame seeds and serve.

1 cup uncooked sprouted short-grain brown rice

Sea salt

1 tablespoon sesame oil

1 garlic clove, minced

1 tablespoon grated or minced fresh ginger

2 small carrots, finely chopped (about ½ cup)

1 cup frozen peas

1 cup frozen corn

1 cup frozen broccoli

1 scallion, chopped

2 tablespoons coconut aminos

2 teaspoons rice vinegar

Sesame seeds, for garnish

PART
TWO

TIER 3
RECIPES

ENTRÉES

OTHER

HUMMUS

SERVES
2

Made from chickpeas, hummus is a must-have for plant-based eating. Use it on sandwiches, as a dip, or—my favorite—to spread on stuffed grape leaves.

// In a high-speed blender or food processor, combine the chickpeas, tahini, lime juice, and salt. Blend until smooth, adding 1 tablespoon of the reserved chickpea can liquid at a time until the desired consistency is reached. Serve immediately or store in an airtight container in the refrigerator for up to 1 week.

1 (15-ounce) can chickpeas, drained (¼ cup liquid from the can reserved) and rinsed

2 tablespoons tahini

Juice of 1 lime

¼ teaspoon sea salt

PART
TWO

TIER 3
RECIPES

ENTRÉES

OTHER

PAGE
284

CUBAN BLACK BEANS

SERVES
4

I grew up on black beans and have always loved them. But it wasn't until college that I realized just what a nutrient powerhouse they are. They're loaded with bone-strengthening calcium, magnesium, manganese, and zinc—nutrients that help regulate blood pressure and insulin levels, prevent heart disease and cancer, and aid digestion. Black beans are also loaded with fiber.

// Put the beans in a large bowl, add cool filtered water to cover, and set aside at room temperature to soak overnight.

// Drain and rinse the beans and transfer them to a large saucepan.

// Add the onion, garlic, bell pepper, cumin, black pepper, vinegar, oregano, salt, and enough water to cover all the ingredients. Bring to a boil, reduce the heat to maintain a simmer and cook, stirring occasionally, for up to 2 hours, until the beans are tender. Add water as needed, $1/2$ cup at a time, to keep the beans simmering.

// Serve immediately, or let cool and store in an airtight container in the refrigerator for 3 to 5 days or in the freezer for up to 8 months.

1 cup dried black beans, rinsed

½ white onion, finely chopped

1 large garlic clove, minced

1 medium green bell pepper, finely chopped

1 tablespoon ground cumin

½ teaspoon freshly ground black pepper

1 tablespoon distilled white vinegar

1 tablespoon dried oregano

1 teaspoon sea salt

PART TWO

—

TIER 3 RECIPES

—

ENTRÉES

—

OTHER

—

PAGE

285

CINNAMON BREAD

MAKES ONE
8 X 4-INCH LOAF

SERVES
12

Here's another delicious creation from the Borges family kitchen! It's naturally sweet, gluten-free, and delicious for breakfast or as a snack.

// Preheat the oven to 350ºF. Line an 8 by 4-inch loaf pan with parchment paper.

// In a large bowl, mix together the applesauce, almond milk, maple syrup, apple, vanilla, and vinegar. Set aside.

// In a separate large bowl, whisk together the gluten-free flour blend, almond flour, flaxseed, chia seeds, baking powder, baking soda, cinnamon, and salt.

// Pour the wet ingredients over the dry ingredients and stir well to combine.

// Pour the batter into the prepared loaf pan and bake for about 50 minutes, or until a toothpick inserted into the center comes out clean. Transfer the pan to a wire rack and let the bread cool in the pan for about 15 minutes, then turn it out onto the rack and let cool completely.

// Slice and serve! The bread can be refrigerated, covered in plastic wrap, for up to 1 week.

1 cup unsweetened applesauce

½ cup sweetened vanilla almond milk

6 tablespoons pure maple syrup

½ apple, peeled, cored, and chopped

1 teaspoon pure vanilla extract

½ teaspoon cider vinegar

1½ cups gluten-free flour blend

½ cup almond flour

1 tablespoon ground flaxseed

1 tablespoon ground chia seeds

2 teaspoons gluten-free baking powder

½ teaspoon baking soda

1 teaspoon ground cinnamon

⅛ teaspoon sea salt

PART
TWO

———

ALL TIERS

———

DESSERTS
AND TREATS

———

PAGE
286

HEMP HEART FRUIT SALAD

SERVES
1

Here's one of my favorite fruit salads. Hemp hearts are loaded with protein and heart-healthy omega-3 fatty acids. The berries are antioxidant champions. Together, they make a perfect meal that's as easy to make as it is delicious and filling.

// In a medium bowl, combine all the berries.

// Add the hemp hearts and orange juice. Toss to coat evenly and serve.

1 cup blueberries

1 cup blackberries

1 cup sliced strawberries

1 cup raspberries

¼ cup hemp hearts

Juice of 1 orange

TIP

Top the salad with your favorite coconut yogurt or almond yogurt for a little extra fuel.

BERRY CHIA PUDDING

SERVES
2

Who doesn't love pudding? Here's a guilt-free take on pudding that incorporates chia seeds, which are loaded with heart-healthy omega-3 fatty acids, vitamins, minerals, antioxidants, and fiber. Enjoy this dish as a dessert or for breakfast.

// In a mason jar or other glass container with a lid, stir together the almond milk and chia seeds until well combined. Cover and refrigerate overnight.

// When ready to serve, divide the pudding between two clean mason jars, alternating with layers of the berries.

2 cups almond milk or other nondairy milk

½ cup chia seeds

1 cup blueberries

1 cup raspberries

1 cup sliced strawberries

PART
TWO

———

ALL TIERS

———

DESSERTS
AND TREATS

———

PAGE
288

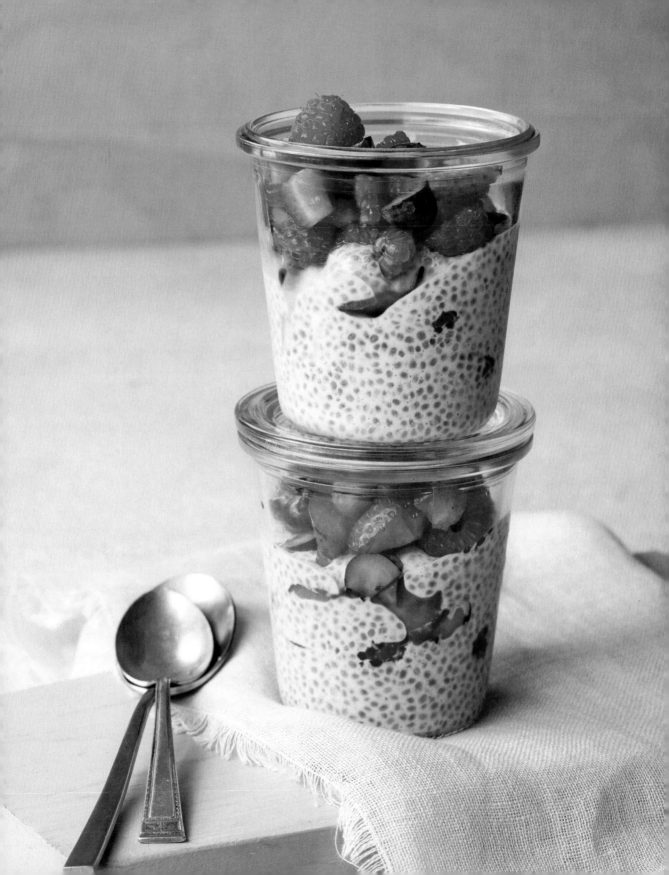

PEANUT BUTTER AND JELLY CHIA PUDDING

SERVES
2

This recipe turns the traditional PB&J sandwich into a tasty pudding that's guaranteed to become a classic on its own. Enjoy this pudding as a dessert or for breakfast.

// In a mason jar or other glass container with a lid, stir together the almond milk and chia seeds until well combined. Cover and refrigerate overnight.

// Combine the berries in a bowl and lightly mash with a fork.

// When ready to serve, divide the pudding between two clean mason jars, alternating with layers of the mashed berries and peanut butter. Top with the peanuts and enjoy!

2 cups almond milk or other nondairy milk

½ cup chia seeds

1½ cups blueberries

1½ cups raspberries

¼ cup crunchy peanut butter

2 tablespoons raw peanuts

PART
TWO

—

ALL TIERS

—

DESSERTS
AND TREATS

—

PAGE
290

PINEAPPLE NICE CREAM

SERVES
2

This is an incredibly creamy tropical treat. It is completely free of dairy and eggs but bursting with pineapple flavor.

2 cups frozen pineapple chunks

½ teaspoon fresh lime juice

// In a high-speed blender, combine the pineapple and lime juice. Blend on low, slowly increasing the speed to high, until smooth and creamy, about 30 seconds. Add water, 1 tablespoon at a time, if needed to facilitate blending.

// Enjoy immediately or pour into an airtight container and freeze until ready to enjoy. It can be kept in the freezer for up to 1 month.

PART
TWO

—

ALL TIERS

—

DESSERTS
AND TREATS

—

PAGE
291

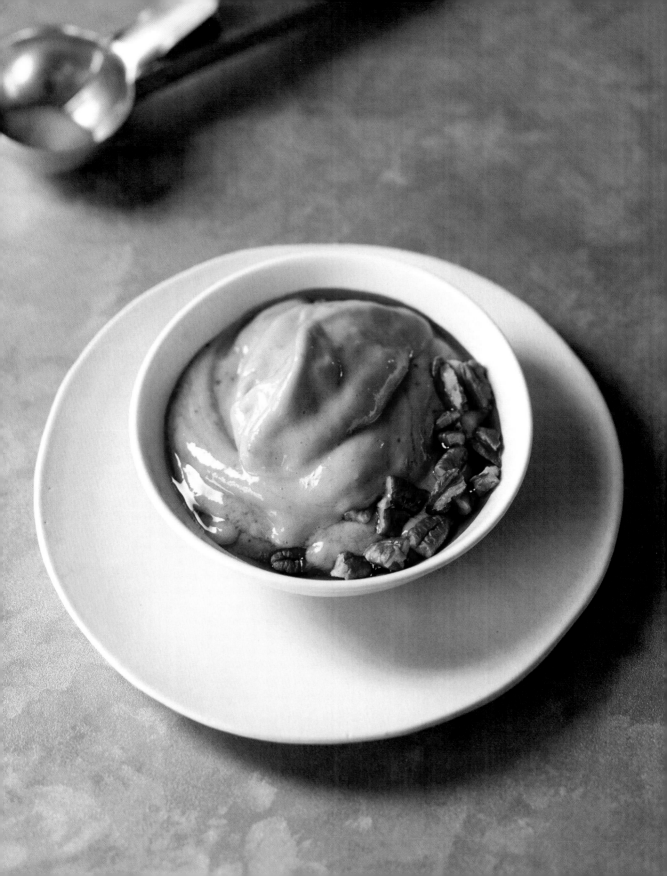

BANANA NICE CREAM BOWL WITH PECANS

SERVES
2

You can easily whip up your own guilt-free ice cream using bananas as a creamy base. The pecans add an extra boost of protein, fiber, vitamins, and minerals.

2 frozen large bananas

⅓ cup raw pecans

¼ cup pure maple syrup

// In a food processor, pulse the frozen bananas until broken down to an ice cream–like texture.

// In a small bowl, stir together the pecans and maple syrup until the nuts are evenly coated.

// Serve the pecans over scoops of the banana nice cream.

TIP

You could use a masticating juicer or high-speed blender to make this recipe in place of the food processor.

PART
TWO

—

ALL TIERS

—

DESSERTS
AND TREATS

—

PAGE
293

WATERMELON ICE POPS

SERVES
4

Here's a fruity, refreshing treat that both kids and adults go for in a big way. Watermelon is the perfect base for these delicious ice pops.

// In a blender or food processor, puree the watermelon cubes until smooth.

// Pour the watermelon puree into ice pop molds, filling each one about two-thirds full.

// Add ice pop sticks and freeze until the pops are firm, about 2 hours.

// Meanwhile, in a blender or food processor, combine the kiwi and maple syrup and blend until smooth.

// Pour the kiwi mixture over the watermelon layer in the molds and freeze at least 4 hours or until solid.

4 cups cubed seedless watermelon

3 kiwifruit, peeled and chopped

1 to 2 tablespoons pure maple syrup (optional)

PART
TWO

———

ALL TIERS

———

DESSERTS
AND TREATS

———

PAGE
294

SORBET

SERVES
2

Sorbet is pure fruit ice cream. Folklore has it that the Roman emperor Nero invented sorbet during the first century AD when he had runners pass buckets of snow from the mountains to his banquet hall, where it was then mixed with honey and wine. You'll be amazed at how easily you can whip up a sorbet in a blender, food processor, or even an ice cream maker using just some frozen fruit and other ingredients you likely have on hand.

// In a high-speed blender or food processor, combine the raspberries and coconut milk and blend until smooth.

// Strain the puree through a fine-mesh sieve into a bowl, pressing it through with a rubber spatula. Discard the seeds in the sieve.

// Stir the maple syrup and vanilla into the puree. Cover and refrigerate for at least 1 hour.

// Transfer the chilled sorbet base to the freezer until frozen, 4 to 6 hours. If it gets too hard, let it soften in the refrigerator prior to serving.

// Scoop into bowls and serve.

2 cups raspberries

½ cup coconut milk (canned unsweetened full fat)

¼ cup pure maple syrup

½ teaspoon pure vanilla extract

TIP

If you are using an ice cream maker, transfer the chilled sorbet base to the machine in the fourth step and follow the manufacturer's instructions to churn it into sorbet.

PART
TWO

ALL TIERS

DESSERTS
AND TREATS

PAGE
295

CONCLUSION
BE THE GREENPRINT

You may have started *The Greenprint* with the intention of improving your own health and well-being. But embracing the plan means that you'll also be improving the planet's health.

Early on, I invited you to take a snapshot of your health before you started the Greenprint program. Now it's time to evaluate the changes you saw and experienced while following the program—things like weight loss; increased energy, endurance, strength, and recovery; and improved health markers like blood pressure, blood sugar, and cholesterol levels. Evaluate other factors, too, such as sleep quality, sex drive, and overall energy. These can also give you black-and-white evidence of the impact the Greenprint is having on you and your life.

I now ask you to take this evaluation one step further—by calculating your personal greenprint using a special tool I created and have made available through 22daysnutrition.com. It gives you concrete evidence of the positive impact your food decisions and lifestyle have on the planet—everything from reducing the size of your carbon footprint to preserving natural resources like fresh water. You can be the change, not only for yourself, but for those around you—and for the world.

This is important. The health of people on earth is declining. Our planet's climate is changing. There is clearly a direct relationship between food choices, human activity, increases in greenhouse gases, and global warming.

It has taken more than two decades for the idea that human activity impacts the environment to become widely accepted by scientists. Most now know that the surge in CO_2 emissions over the last thirty years is directly related to the burning of fossil fuels. Global warming is an evidence-based model that reflects the influence of humans on the earth's climate and on the balance of its ecosystems.

Expanding your greenprint goes beyond making plant-based food choices, although this action is the most important one you can take in saving the planet. Buy locally grown food. This not only improves health, but also decreases the amount of transportation fuel. Go to a farmers' market instead of the supermarket to purchase local produce and take public transportation instead of driving. Grow a vegetable garden, plant trees, recycle, compost, and avoid buying so many packaged products.

Calculating your greenprint gives you insight into the way your everyday actions affect your health and the planet, and the steps you can take to change that impact.

My mission is to introduce you to simple, actionable ways that you can make your greenprint count, beginning with choosing a 100 percent plant-based diet. As you shift your habits, you'll begin to see how one person—you—can make a huge difference in the world. I will do my part to expand my personal greenprint, and I hope you will, too.

ACKNOWLEDGMENTS

I am incredibly grateful for the amazing people in my life and for all the wonderful people I have yet to meet.

A heartfelt thank-you to my dear friend Raymond Garcia, for daring to dream with me and believing in the possibilities.

To Diana Baroni and my friends at the Crown Publishing Group: Thank you for your vision and creativity.

To my friend Maggie Greenwood-Robinson: A huge thank-you for all your help bringing this idea to life.

To my agent, Byrd Leavell: Your enthusiasm is infectious and your kindness is inspiring. Thank you for your trust and friendship.

To Jay and BB: I'm forever grateful for your kindness and friendship, and love you immensely for it.

To Mami, Angelo, Alfredo, Jennifer, and the rest of my family: I feel fortunate to be on this journey with you, and love you with all my heart.

Last, to Marilyn, Mila, Maximo, Mateo, and Marco Jr.: My love for you is boundless, and life with you is so beautiful.

RESOURCES

There's a lot of information out there about vegan and plant-based eating—so much that it can be overwhelming. I've culled this information down to a few resources that will be the most helpful—and not bog you down.

22 DAYS NUTRITION:
22daysnutrition.com

22 DAYS MEAL PLANNER:
mealplanner.22daysnutrition.com

BARNARD MEDICAL CENTER:
pcrm.org/barnard-medical-center

BLUE ZONES: bluezones.com

THE CHINA STUDY:
nutritionstudies.org/the-china-study

EAT DRINK VEGAN: eatdrinkvegan.com

DR. ESSELSTYN: dresselstyn.com/site

FARM SANCTUARY: farmsanctuary.org

KATHY FRESTON: kathyfreston.com

DR. FUHRMAN: drfuhrman.com/get-started

HAPPY COW: happycow.net

DR. JOEL KAHN: drjoelkahn.com

LIVE KINDLY: livekindly.co

MERCY FOR ANIMALS: mercyforanimals.org

NUTRITION FACTS: nutritionfacts.org

DR. DEAN ORNISH: ornish.com

PCRM: pcrm.org

PETA: peta.org

JULIE PIATT: srimati.com

PLANT-BASED NEWS: plantbasednews.org

RICH ROLL: richroll.com

SEED FOOD AND WINE FESTIVAL:
seedfoodandwine.com

THRIVE MAGAZINE: mythrivemag.com

VEGNEWS: vegnews.com

SELECTED REFERENCES

Abdulla, M., et al. "Nutrient Intake and Health Status of Vegans. Chemical Analyses of Diets Using the Duplicate Portion Sampling Technique." *American Journal of Clinical Nutrition* 34 (1981): 2464–77.

Acito, M., and M. Maron. Holy Name Greenprint Study, May 2018.

Adan, A. "Cognitive Performance and Dehydration." *Journal of the American College of Nutrition* 31 (2012): 71–78.

Afshin, A., et al. "Consumption of Nuts and Legumes and Risk of Incident Ischemic Heart Disease, Stroke, and Diabetes: A Systematic Review and Meta-Analysis." *American Journal of Clinical Nutrition* 100 (2014): 278–88.

Arem, H., et al. "Leisure Time Physical Activity and Mortality: A Detailed Pooled Analysis of the Dose-Response Relationship." *JAMA Internal Medicine* 175 (2015): 959–67.

Barnard, N. "Fiber Is the Key to Good Health." *Dr. Barnard's Blog* (blog), Physician's Committee for Responsible Medicine (February 18, 2015); pcrm.org/nbBlog/index.php/fiber-is-the-key-to-good-health.

Baroni, L., et al. "Evaluating the Environmental Impact of Various Dietary Patterns Combined with Different Food Production Systems." *European Journal of Clinical Nutrition* 61 (2007): 279–86.

Bhupathiraju, S. N., et al. "Quantity and Variety in Fruit and Vegetable Intake and Risk of Coronary Heart Disease." *American Journal of Clinical Nutrition* 98 (2013): 1514–23.

Boschmann, M., et al. "Water-Induced Thermogenesis." *Journal of Clinical Endocrinology and Metabolism* 88 (2003): 6015–19.

Darmadi-Blackberry, I., et al. "Legumes: The Most Important Dietary Predictor of Survival in Older People of Different Ethnicities." *Asia Pacific Journal of Clinical Nutrition* 13 (2004): 217–20.

Devore, E. E., et al. "Dietary Fat Intake and Cognitive Decline in Women with Type 2 Diabetes." *Diabetes Care* 32 (2009): 635–40.

Du, H., et al. "Fresh Fruit Consumption and Major Cardiovascular Disease in China." *New England Journal of Medicine* 374 (2016): 1332–43.

Esselstyn, C. B., et al. "A Way to Reverse CAD?" *Journal of Family Practice* 63 (2014): 356–64b.

Fry, P. S., and D. L. Debats. "Perfectionism and the Five-Factor Personality Traits as Predictors of Mortality in Older Adults." *Journal of Health Psychology* 14 (2009): 513–24.

Giem, P., W. L. Beeson, and G. E. Fraser. "The Incidence of Dementia and Intake of Animal Products: Preliminary Findings from the Adventist Health Study." *Neuroepidemiology* 12 (1993): 28–36.

Grant, W. B. "Using Multicountry Ecological and Observational Studies to Determine Dietary Risk Factors for Alzheimer's disease." *Journal of the American College of Nutrition* 35 (2016): 476–89.

Hanson, A. J., et al. "Effect of Apolipoprotein E Genotype and Diet on Apolipoprotein E Lipidation and Amyloid Peptides: Randomized Clinical Trial." *JAMA Neurology* 70 (2013): 972–80.

Hernando-Requejo, V. "Nutrition and Cognitive Impairment." *Nutricion Hospitalaria* 33 (2016): 346.

Jacobs, D. R., et al. "Fiber from Whole Grains, But Not Refined Grains, Is Inversely Associated with All-Cause Mortality in Older Women: The Iowa Women's Health Study." *Journal of the American College of Nutrition* 19 (2000): 326S–330S.

Jakse, B., et al. "Effects of an Ad Libitum Consumed Low-Fat Plant-Based Diet Supplemented with Plant-Based Meal Replacements on Body Composition Indices." *BioMed Research International* 2017 (March 28, 2017). doi.org/10.1155/2017/9626390.

Kaczmarczyk, M. M., M. J. Miller, and G. G. Freund. "The Health Benefits of Dietary Fiber: Beyond the Usual Suspects of Type 2 Diabetes Mellitus, Cardiovascular Disease and Colon Cancer." *Metabolism* 61 (2012): 1058–66.

Kahn, H. S., L. M. Tatham, and C. W. Heath Jr.. "Contrasting Factors Associated with Abdominal and Peripheral Weight Gain Among Adult Women." *International Journal of Obesity and Related Metabolic Disorders* 21 (1997): 903–11.

Kahn, J. "The Environmental Impact of Eating Vegan for Just One Day." drjoelkahn.com, May 19, 2017.

Kleiner, S. M. "Water: An Essential but Overlooked Nutrient." *Journal of the American Dietetic Association* 99 (1999): 200–6.

Kouvari, M., et al. "Exclusive Olive Oil Consumption and 10-Year (2004–2014) Acute Coronary Syndrome Incidence Among Cardiac Patients: The GREECS Observational Study." *Journal of Human Nutrition and Dietetics* 29 (2016): 354–62.

Le, L. T., and J. Sabaté. "Beyond Meatless, the Health Effects of Vegan Diets: Findings from the Adventist Cohorts." *Nutrients* 6 (2014): 2131–47.

Mattson, M. P., V. D. Longo, and M. Harvie. "Impact of Intermittent Fasting on Health and Disease Processes." *Ageing Research Reviews* 39 (2017): 46–58.

McKeown, N. M., et al. "Whole-Grain Intake and Cereal Fiber Are Associated with Lower Abdominal Adiposity in Older Adults." *Journal of Nutrition* 139 (2009): 1950–55.

Messina, V. "Nutritional and Health Benefits of Dried Beans." *American Journal of Clinical Nutrition* 100 (2014): 437S–442S.

Mishra, B. N. "Secret of Eternal Youth; Teaching from the Centenarian Hot Spots ('Blue Zones')." *Indian Journal of Community Medicine* 34 (2009): 273–75.

Ogata, K., et al. "The Effectiveness of Cognitive Behavioral Therapy with Mindfulness and an Internet Intervention for Obesity: A Case Series." *Frontiers in Nutrition* 5 (2018): 56.

O'Reilly, G. A., et al. "Mindfulness-Based Interventions for Obesity-Related Eating Behaviors: A Literature Review." *Obesity Reviews* 15 (2014): 453–61.

Orlich, M. J., and G. E. Fraser. "Vegetarian Diets in the Adventist Health Study 2: A Review of Initial Published Findings." *American Journal of Clinical Nutrition* 100 (2014): 353–58.

Rickman, J. C., D. M. Barrett, and C. M. Bruhn. "Review—Nutritional Comparison of Fresh, Frozen and Canned Fruits and Vegetables. Part 1. Vitamins C and B and Phenolic Compounds." *Journal of the Science of Food and Agriculture* 87 (2007): 930–44.

Rogerson, D. "Vegan Diets: Practical Advice for Athletes and Exercisers." *Journal of the International Society of Sports Nutrition* 13 (2017): 14–36.

Rolls, B. J. "Dietary Strategies for Weight Management." *Nestlé Nutrition Institute Workshop series* 73 (2012): 37–48.

Rosell, M., et al. "Weight Gain over 5 Years in 21,966 Meat-Eating, Fish-Eating, Vegetarian, and Vegan Men and Women in EPIC-Oxford." *International Journal of Obesity* 30 (2006): 1389–96.

Satija, A., et al. "Healthful and Unhealthful Plant-Based Diets and the Risk of Coronary Heart Disease in U.S. Adults." *Journal of the American College of Cardiology* 70 (2017): 411–22.

Schmidt, J. A., et al. "Metabolic Profiles of Male Meat Eaters, Fish Eaters, Vegetarians, and Vegans From the EPIC-Oxford Cohort." *American Journal of Clinical Nutrition* 102 (2015): 1518–26.

Sears, M. E., K. J. Kerr, and R. I. Bray. "Arsenic, Cadmium, Lead, and Mercury in Sweat: A Systematic Review." *Journal of Environmental and Public Health* 2012 (February 22, 2012). doi.org/10.1155/2012/184745.

Seimon, R. V., et al. "Do Intermittent Diets Provide Physiological Benefits Over Continuous Diets for Weight Loss? A Systematic Review of Clinical Trials." *Molecular and Cellular Endocrinology* 418, part 2 (2015): 153–72.

Sin, N. L. "The Protective Role of Positive Well-Being in Cardiovascular Disease: Review of Current Evidence, Mechanisms, and Clinical Implications." *Current Cardiology Reports* 18 (2016): 106.

Sinha, R., et al. "Meat Intake and Mortality: A Prospective Study of Over Half a Million People." *Archives of Internal Medicine* 169 (2009): 562–71.

Smith-Splangler, C., et al. "Are Organic Foods Safer or Healthier Than Conventional Alternatives? A Systematic Review." *Annals of Internal Medicine* 157 (2012): 348–66.

Song, M., et al. "Association of Animal and Plant Protein Intake with All-Cause and Cause-Specific Mortality." *JAMA Internal Medicine* 176 (2016): 1453–63.

Spence, J. D. "Controlling Resistant Hypertension." *Stroke and Vascular Neurology* 24 (2018): 69–75.

Tripathi, V. "Organic Farming: A New Avenue for Rural Entrepreneurs for Sustainable Business." *International Journal of Education and Management Studies*, #6:1 (2016): 8.

Turner-McGrievy, G. M., et al. "Comparative Effectiveness of Plant-Based Diets for Weight Loss: A Randomized Controlled Trial of Five Different Diets." *Nutrition* 31 (2015): 350–58.

Zong, G., et al. "Whole Grain Intake and Mortality from All Causes, Cardiovascular Disease, and Cancer: A Meta-Analysis of Prospective Cohort Studies." *Circulation* 133 (2016): 2370–80.

INDEX

ABOUT THE AUTHOR

MARCO BORGES //// is an exercise physiologist, the founder of 22 Days Nutrition, a *New York Times*-bestselling author, and a plant-based living advocate. Passionate about guiding people to develop healthier lifestyles, he has spent more than twenty years as a lifestyle coach, touring the world to empower others with tools for ultimate wellness. Author of *The 22-Day Revolution*, *The 22-Day Revolution Cookbook*, and *Power Moves*, he lives in Miami with his wife and their three sons and daughter.

The book that will finally give you the tools, recipes, and systems to catalyze *LASTING TRANSFORMATION* into your life, from one of the most educated and impactful leaders in the wellness space today.

–JULIE PIATT, coauthor of *The Plantpower Way*

The Greenprint is the *BLUEPRINT* to build your healthiest and most satisfying life. You are twenty-two days and twenty-two rules away from finding out that you can feel good every day.

–JOEL KAHN, MD, FACC, author, *The Plant-Based Solution*

A MUST-READ for anyone wanting power over their health. The benefits are amazing, achievable, and totally within your control.

–MICHAEL MARON, president and CEO, Holy Name Medical Center, Teaneck, New Jersey

The Greenprint is the book all *JUNK FOOD EATERS,* like myself, have been waiting for . . . a guide to the healthy side of living.

–MARY MATTERN, author of *Nom Yourself*

With the *GREENPRINT MOVEMENT,* Marco Borges will help older and younger generations consume and demand more plant-based foods, prevent and reverse disease, and preserve our beautiful planet.

–JOHN SALLEY, NBA champion and wellness advocate